This is ^Not the End Beautiful Friend

*Steps to Help Someone at the End-of-Life Maintain Peace
and Dignity... While Providing Guidance and
Reassurance to Everyone Else*

Rich Nisbet

This is Not the End Beautiful Friend

Published by:

Rp Robertson Publishing™
www.RobertsonPublishing.com

Printed in the USA and UK on acid-free paper.

TABLE of CONTENTS

Heroes

Those that have demonstrated the courage to use the steps outlined in this book are real heroes.

In the following pages you are going to read the stories of individuals who took it upon themselves to observe that someone close to them was in need of help... a special kind of help... the kind of help that brings aid to someone who is dying.

Having the care and bravery to look, ask, learn and administer some simple instructions that bring comfort and reassurance to a loved one who is at the end of his or her life, is extremely admirable, to say the least.

I would never have even thought to research and write about this whole subject, unless over a decade ago, a client of mine hadn't asked my advice on how he could help his dying grandmother.

This book is intended to furnish knowledge and direction to those individuals who desire to provide assistance to someone at the end of life. You can also refer this information to another who may need help in providing comfort to a family member or a close friend.

Or, just read it for the subject matter and stories it reveals.

The main contents contain how this end of life program was developed, the theory behind it, the different examples of how it has been utilized, some effective steps to follow, some types of strange phenomena that might be encountered and finally, thoughts to consider regarding how to look at death *and* life.

The primary goal is to help someone who is dying, pass away as peacefully and with as much dignity as possible. One other thing, because some of these topics around death are often shied away from and because of all the implications that come with it, I have tried to keep this compilation of guidelines and the subject matter itself as "light" as possible. It is not to minimize what others may be feeling, but I will attempt to detail everything so it is easy to read, digest and apply.

Here we go...

One more day

One more time

One more sunset, maybe I'd be satisfied

But then again

I know what it would do

Leave me wishing still, for one more day with you

*~ **Diamond Rio***

Section One

A Very Good Place To Start

The Story

1.

From the Beginning

Emotional loss can have a very painful, gripping and devastating effect on a person.

Losing family members, loss of friends, death of a loved one, pets running away or growing old, divorce, losing a career, having to give up a home you love, abuse, feeling unappreciated or unacknowledged and ramifications from prolonged illness or injury, are examples of events most everyone will eventually have to face and deal with at some point in their life.

Even the loss of one's identity, like when the children have grown and left the house, the role of mother or father is no longer the same as it was when the kids were young. That void of purpose can be overwhelming.

Because of all this, the idea of death seems to be a subject filled with apprehension and fear, due to the severity of losing your entire life and everything and everyone connected with it.

This became evident when I launched a podcast series entitled, *"It's the Question"*. In each episode a universal type of question is proposed so listeners can email in their answers, experiences and stories. It's a forum I call a "virtual campfire". It's for anyone who wants to discuss the deeper questions about our existence here in this universe.

Well, in one of these podcast episodes, we asked the question, *"What happens when you die?"* Here are some answers listeners wrote in:

"I hope it's not painful."

"That's a scary question."

"I don't want to think about it."

Losing one's life is obviously an occurrence people try to stay away from and not even talk about. Yet it is something everyone will go through.

So, how is it that I happened to learn about this and figure out some simple steps to provide aid to those who are dying?

To tell the truth, I kind of stumbled into it.

In my private practice, as a counselor/coach for individuals, business owners, couples and kids, I'm often required to provide assistance to those that have experienced some level of grief and loss in their lives.

It is a subject that I had to study, approach and learn how to alleviate for a variety of people of all different ages and backgrounds.

(For reasons of confidentiality, I will not be including the identities of those individuals who have shared their experiences with me for this book.)

Over a decade ago, a client of mine asked if I could advise him on how to deal with his grandmother who was in the hospital. He told me she was not doing well, everyone was concerned, she'd been in this horrible condition for weeks, and the doctors said there was no hope for any medical procedure to remedy her condition. She was dying but couldn't die.

I told him I'd have to think about it.

That evening, I started out by listing all the possible situations that people face in normal life where there is an extreme loss or threat of loss. Here are a few examples I came up with:

- A husband/father, who is supporting a family, loses his job because a larger company is acquiring the organization he worked for.
- A wife finding out her husband is having an affair.
- A hurricane wiping out a home with all its possessions.
- A sports figure who, because of age, is forced to retire and so no longer has the camaraderie of his teammates or adulation from his fans.
- Your child walking out the door to report for active duty in a country thousands of miles away.

I then wrote down what effects these types of losses might have on someone:

- What amounts of overwhelm would be present?
- What emotions would he or she be feeling?
- What fears?

- What other people will be influenced by the loss?
- What planning will need to occur as to what should be done?
- Who should he or she talk to about it?
- What about the parents, in-laws or children affected? How should they be treated and consoled?

I then listed ideas for what a coach could possibly provide:

- What should be done to bring assistance?
- What should be avoided that would only add more confusion?
- What reassurance could be given?
- What kind of direction or counseling would be most effective in alleviating the gripping emotion that loss can hold on a person?

In other words, how do you provide a means to help move life forward again?

After I listed out all these different scenarios, I wrote out what types of counseling tools and coaching techniques I've utilized in the past on others with similar losses.

The original list I came up with looked something like this:

1. Ask how they are feeling, listen fully, and let them know you understand.
2. Establish that help is possible.
3. Find out what they are afraid might happen or the possible consequences due to the loss. Explain that you'll help them figure out some solutions that they consider doable.

4. List whom he or she needs to talk to and what they will say to each person.

5. Get some details as to how they will approach their immediate family and urge them to be as open as possible.

6. Work out some simple plans based on everything you've gone over and set a time you will meet again to review the progress.

7. Utilize grief counseling and anything else applicable to remove frozen emotions and any debilitating decisions to help get life moving again.

I then listed out everything I could imagine my client would need to do to help his grandmother and what would make sense as to how to possibly help provide some shred of relief from the inevitable.

Here is a basic list of steps I advised:

1. When you arrive at the hospital, make sure that the room and environment is as stable, uncluttered and calm as possible.

2. Try to spend the initial visit with your grandma alone, without others in the room, so as not to be distracted or interrupted.

3. If verbal speaking is too difficult for her, workout some type of communication method, ABC word-charts, squeeze my hands, blinking etc.

4. Have her look at and touch things in the room until she seems calmer than when you started.

5. Ask if she has her attention on anything or needs

something you can help her with. Make a list and tell her you'll take care if everything.

6. If applicable, discuss the Spirit-Mind-Body idea to point out that there may be hope for continuing after her body has ceased.

7. Let me know how it goes and any changes you notice in her physical condition and emotional state.

Well, he did it. He went where she was; spent a couple hours with her doing some of these steps, and the results were pretty remarkable. Here is his story:

"When I arrived at the hospital, my grandma was lying in the bed, shaking, incoherent, her extremities were purple, her tongue was out of her mouth and she couldn't speak. Apparently, she'd been like this for several days.

I told her I was there to help her, and I asked the rest of the people in the room (my mom, my aunt and the nurse) to please give me a few minutes alone with grandma, which they did.

Because grandma couldn't speak, we worked out a simple system to communicate without verbal words. I instructed her to squeeze my hand once for no and twice for yes. It worked!

I then began asking her to notice things around the room. At first, I did it wrong but soon realized that I needed to find objects closer to her, which helped. We did this for some minutes until it appeared she was a bit more settled down from the anxiety she had been in.

I then continued with the next steps of the program, and around step 5 or 6, I noticed the color in her skin returned to normal, her tongue went back in her mouth, she could now speak somewhat, and that look of total fear was gone. It was a miracle. We talked a bit about what was happening with her and what she might expect.

When I had my mom, my aunt and the nurse return to the room, they were completely amazed at the change in grandma. She was talking again with them and was no longer in pain and showed no more anxiety. They couldn't believe the huge change after just that short period of time.

Grandma passed away peacefully that very evening.

The fact that we all could spend her last hours together in a serene and loving way was the best sendoff we could have ever hoped for.

I'll never forget that day."

* * *

I figured this might have been an isolated instance, a fluke or a coincidence, but soon the word got out and I had others asking me what to do about someone in their life who was dying. I continued to coach them, utilizing those same successful steps, while at the same time, adding others when applicable and refining the ones I'd previously outlined.

In every instance the results kept coming back as favorable, supportive and helpful. Those individuals to whom the steps were administered, each one, passed away in a peaceful and dignified manner on that same day or a day or two later.

They were finally able to "let go". Their last hours in this life, and their passing, went off as serene and as comfortable as could be imagined, and the memories for the living, regarding the death of his or her loved one, were peaceful and loving as well.

I know people have been dying for hundreds of thousands of years without using the information in these pages. I also know that death has generally been a subject that has been shied away from, and as a result, there has been a relatively limited amount of words written about it.

Dr. Christopher Kerr explained in a TedX talk entitled, *"I See Dead People – Dreams and Visions of the Dying"* (2015 in Buffalo, New York): *"Medical training is how to defy death, and when you can't defy it, you deny it, in whole or in part."*

In his book, *"Being Mortal"*, Dr. Atul Gawande details how his studies taught him how to save lives with operations and surgeries, but he never learned how to communicate about death with his patients and their loved ones.

Nurses and hospice personnel probably have the greatest wealth of knowledge and experience in this area. They normally have a very intimate relationship with people near the end of their lives and have seen more than most regarding what to expect.

All I can say is, the steps you will read here have seemed to genuinely help those individuals who were at the end of their life, as well as their associated family and friends.

2.

An Overview of What's to Come

Consider this a "how-to" book. It is also a compilation of what many others have said around the subject of life and death as it applies to what I have experienced. I've tried to include only enough information to explain the important details behind each of the steps that have helped bring aid to someone at the end of his or her life.

The chapters on Identity, Secrets, Hard Core Soft Skills, The Human Spirit, Paranormal Phenomena, etc., are a few of the subjects that have been touched on just enough to be relevant to what you'll need to be effective. I've referenced other people who have covered some of these related subjects in books, lectures and videos. I've also attempted to provide some background knowledge, so that when you apply the various procedures herein, you'll have a bit more reference as to why these steps can work.

Since the subject of death is the other side of life, you will hopefully gain a deeper awareness of yourself and your own existence now, while learning how to help someone else pass away peacefully.

3.

Coach

In a game of sports, the coach is there to give direction and confidence so his players can hopefully win the game. A minister, rabbi or priest is there to help the parishioner find the faith that will give them purpose here on earth and in the after-life. A doctor or nurse is there to help that patient get well. A counselor is there to listen and help the patient get some relief from trauma or confusion, and thus face life easier. A life coach is there to help the client live a more enriched existence with less effort.

But what if the person in front of you is dying?

What steps will you take? What are you going to advise, suggest or ask of him or her? What outcome are you hoping to achieve?

The goal of living a better life or getting well isn't the point anymore. The purpose needs to shift to "helping a person who is facing physical mortality".

"Coach" is what I am calling the individual helping the person at the end of life. As a coach you'll be providing aid and resolving any unfinished communications. Giving reassurance and help in coming to terms with any regrets they are hanging onto. Reducing fears and anxieties.

Allowing them to know that their worries are being taken care of. Helping him or her to transition and move on to whatever the next chapter holds for them in this universe.

You as a coach are providing a closure to this life so the dying person can "let go" with less trepidation, fewer struggles and an acceptance of the same life cycle that everyone is part of, the end of which, we all will eventually have to face.

No matter your belief in what happens after a body dies, the cycle of death carries with it fear, uncertainty, loss of possessions, loss of friends, loss of family and loss of identity. This is what you're there to coach them through with compassion, direction and reassurance.

4.

Belief Versus Science

There has always been this point where science ends and spirituality begins.

Science continues to attempt to push further and further into proving how the universe and life were created. Albert Einstein and Stephen Hawking were extremely intelligent and courageous individuals who kept asking "why" regarding the bigger questions to our existence.

Religion often gives comfort and hope that there is something beyond the scope of what is in front of our faces. Belief in something higher and more profound than our physical experience on earth, in these little human bodies, can help provide a calmness that it will all be okay.

Belief is a whole subject in itself. Quite powerful to say the least.

When it comes to death of the body, it is anyone's guess as to what happens next.

I am making no claims regarding religion or science. I only know that with a good heart, some common sense and the application of the steps you'll read herein, it is possible to help people at the end of their life.

Section Two

CHECKLIST OF STEPS

For further reference regarding a particular step, note the page number next to it, which will then take you to the corresponding chapter that provides further instructions and background information to help you administer that step.

5.

Preparation

1. To familiarize yourself with the various recommendations and possible scenarios you may run into, read as much of this book as you can.

2. If possible, establish the condition and current status of the dying person.

3. Look over the steps below and write a general order you feel will be the best way to apply them. (pg. 157)

4. If applicable, establish who you'll need to coordinate with, perhaps the daughter, minister, doctor etc. (pg. 156)

5. This next step can be done by a family member who would know how to put this together: (pg. 72)

   a. Arrange a group email list of all the friends and family across the world that knows the person who is now dying.

   b. Create and send an email to everyone on that list, asking them to write and email you a one page letter that can be read to the dying person.

   c. Have them say whatever they want to say, what they are thankful for, humorous events that they've shared together, and how they have been helped because of their mutual association.

d. Tell them to keep their own emotions of loss out of it so as not to burden the dying person, who can't do anything about the situation.

e. Get these letters printed out and compiled in a book. (An office supply store can help with this.) The book can be called "*Letters to* [dying person's first name]", with a picture of him or her on the cover if desired.

f. Arrange to start getting these letters read to the person each day, a few pages at a time.

6.

Helping the Person at the End of Life

1. Establish why you're there.

2. Attempt to be alone with them if possible. (pg. 170)

3. Stay clear of your "associative identity" as much as you can while administering these steps. (pg. 29)

4. Use a talk relay if applicable. (pg. 173)

5. Put order into the room environment if needed. (pg. 170)

6. Human Touch techniques (pg. 46)

7. Stability techniques. (pg. 49)

8. Establish a future. Ask about their beliefs concerning the after-life. (pg. 52)

9. Let them know at any point they want to let go, it's okay. (pg. 169)

10. List out the things they have attention on completing or are causing them concern. (pg. 57)

11. List out messages or what they want said to individuals they have attention on. (pg. 59)

12. Secrets technique as applicable. (pg. 33)

13. Progressive directive regarding "Prevent Leaving". (pg. 49)

14. Remove yourself from the room periodically and ensure others do the same. (pg. 65)

15. You can do steps 6 & 7 daily.

16. Read from the "Letters to ____" book daily.

17. Continue to help them with what they need.

18. End-off each visit at any positive change. Don't push it. (pg. 136)

7.

Everyone Else

1. Tell everyone to quit asking the dying person not to die. (pg. 169)

2. If possible, have the dying person deliver their last communications to those that will need it, especially kids and grandkids. (pg. 76)

3. Answer people's questions but do not violate any confidentiality you've established with the dying person.

4. Make sure everyone leaves the room for periods of time in case the dying person wants to be alone when he or she decides it's time to "let go". (pg. 65)

5. Be a stable influence for everyone.

8.

After the Memorial

1. Reassure anyone as you best you can.

2. Ensure everyone is offered the "Letters to ____" book.

3. Offer or refer those that need it to Grief Counseling. (pg. 181)

4. Suggest that people discuss their own wishes and arrangements for what they want at the end of their own life by working it all in writing for future peace of mind. (pg. 41)

5. Refer those that need it to the "Words of Love" section in this book, for advice from the elderly as to how to live out the remaining days of one's life in a meaningful way. (pg. 185)

Section Three

THE REAL RELATION,
THE UNDERLYING THEME

Philosophies – Ideas – Examples - Experiences.

9.

For Whom the Bell Tolls

One of the biggest mysteries of life is death. Everyone is going to have to deal with death at some point... even your own.

This information is for anyone of any faith, belief, non-belief, spiritual conviction, or life/death orientation. These guidelines can be adapted and applied to anyone at the end of his or her life. It doesn't matter if the person considers themselves Christian, Atheist, Buddhist, Jewish, Hindu, Islamic, New Age, Mormon, scientific, unscientific, or just a plain human being.

Most all religions in the world are based on a promise of life after body death. The bestselling book in the world is the Bible, a book about the things you need to think about and prepare for, and so hopefully achieve an infinite awareness of yourself after your body has expired.

John 3:16 *"For God so loved the world that He gave His one and only Son, that everyone who believes in Him shall not perish but have eternal life"*.

Eternal life is a long time.

It is not anyone's place to tell somebody what to believe

about the after-life, and that especially applies to someone who is dying. As a matter of fact, one of the most important steps to take is to establish what the dying person believes is going to happen when they pass away, and make sure to align all assistance to that belief.

Here are some facts on death. The average lifespan for a human body, at the time of this writing, is 79 years. The news is a little better for women and a little worse for men. Life expectancy for females is 81.2 years and for males it's 76.4 years. [1]

Take 79 years, multiply it by 12 months and you'll find that from birth to body death, you only have 948 months of life as who you are, in the body you are now occupying. 948 months of existence? Is that it? Really?

If you want to really freak yourself out, subtract your age now from 79, multiply it by 12 and you'll see the number of months you've got left.

As portrayed in the movie "Spinal Tap", when the English musicians are staring at the grave of their mentor, Elvis Presley, Nigel quietly sighed and said, *"It really puts perspective on things doesn't it?"* David, the other guitarist, then blurts out, *"Yeah! Too much f**king perspective!"*

The body is going to die. Then what?

Here is what a few of the major religions of the world believe regarding what happens after death of a body:

Hinduism - Reincarnation. Hindus believe in the rebirth and reincarnation of souls. The souls are immortal and imperishable. [2]

Christianity - Heaven or Hell and/or Purgatory.

Islam - Movement through a separate dimension of existence.

Buddhism - Bardo, in Tibetan Buddhism, a state of existence between death and rebirth, varying in length according to a person's conduct in life and manner of, or age at death. [3]

Judaism - Heaven or Reincarnation (Opinions vary).

Mormon - Spirit and body will be reunited in a perfect, immortal state.

New Age / Spiritualism - Opinions vary.

Atheists - You're gone man, gone.

Most all of these doctrines feel that the quality of your after-life will be dependent on how you've lived your life here on earth. Karma.

Asking about the beliefs and hopes regarding what is going to happen when the body is no longer living is something that can be discussed, as it is probably front and center in the mind of the person on his or her deathbed.

And do not assume that just because grandma has been attending a certain church every Sunday for the last 85 years, that she believes everything she has been told. If she does, fine, but I have talked with several people who secretly have not agreed with all the dogma in their particular religion but still enjoyed being part of their parish or temple for the comfort, support and friendships that a group can provide.

Once it has been established what their beliefs and hopes actually are, the steps you'll apply to help them can be aligned to achieving those purposes. Even an Atheist, who believes it will be "lights out" at body death, will still want his family and friends to be able to carry-on their lives without too much grief. *"Okay grandpa. You told me you hope your kids and grandkids will be okay, so tell me what you want me to relay to everyone."*

If the dying person thinks they are probably going to Hell, ask them what they have done to make them feel that way. In this light, a listening ear may be helpful in providing some relief from the burdens of past guilt.

If they believe they are going to a Heaven, find out if there is anything you can help them with now to make that happen. Do not place judgment. Tailor your actions to fit their faith and help them move closer to achieving their hopes for the after-life.

10.

Identity

*"The true value of a human being is determined
primarily by the measure and the sense in which
he has attained liberation from the Self"*

(Albert Einstein)

The word "personality" comes from the Latin root word
"persona'" which means, "mask". Who you consider you
are, in other words your personality, is a mask that you are
showing and sharing with the world.

When you identify yourself as something, a father, a
mother, a teacher, a doctor, a business owner, a Catholic, a
Democrat, a musician, a daughter etc., each of these identities carry with them certain parameters. Certain rules,
morals, what's right and wrong and "How I am supposed
to think and act".

At the end of life, the realization that this identity or personality will also end can be an upsetting reality for a person. So much has been wrapped up in supporting and
asserting this identity. Identity gives purpose. Identity
provides a reason for existence. Without an identity, there
is "nothing", a lonely proposition.

There could never be an argument without identities involved. Each identity "knows" what is right and what is wrong and thus a clash is possible. Happiness carries the same formula. What makes one identity happy is not necessarily true for another one. Identity makes us all "individuals" with all the pros and cons that go along with it.

Identities give us pain and pleasure, in other words, Life.

On the other side of this there is a freedom associated with not relying on an identity to define yourself. It appears that many of the religious teachings are around this concept. *"Turn the other cheek,"* means, get off your own opinion and see the situation from another, more expansive point of view. Quit looking only through the eyes of that one identity you have assumed.

With death of the body, comes a "death" of the identities that person took-on and lived. Each identity has certain needs, interests, responsibilities and areas of control. An identity affects and influences all the other people associated with that identity: wife, husband, son, daughter, grandma, grandpa, mom, dad, sister, brother, uncle, aunt, cousin, niece, nephew, friend, coworker, acquaintance etc.

We look to each of these labels as something that supports and aids us in our lives, so when death approaches one of our loved ones, who represented an identity we associate ourselves with, our own sense of stability gets threatened. *"How will I carry on without that association?" "What will happen to me when she is gone?" "A part of me dies with him."*

This goes both ways when you are dealing with and

coaching someone at the end of life. First of all, if you are family or friends with the person who is dying, you'll have to keep that identity out of it as much as possible. Putting too much of your "associative personality" (son, daughter, friend, etc.) into these coaching steps will add an additional stress factor and make it more difficult for the dying person to eventually let go.

Of course, you can't deny your associations or pretend your relationship doesn't exist, but you should approach these coaching steps as being "someone there to help". *"Mom, I've asked everyone else to leave the room for now because I am going to help you through all this. Tell me what you have your attention on at the house that you'd like me to take care of?"* is the attitude that will help your mom more than you getting into how much you'll miss her, what a great mom she was or how hard it's going to be on you when she's gone.

Make sure to be aware of these separate identities when applying these steps.

In some writings I've studied, one recommendation, directed to healthcare and social service professionals regarding caring for the elderly, was: *"Detach emotionally but practice compassion".* [4]

Let everyone else become aware that they shouldn't burden the dying person with how hard his or her eventual departure will be on them. I don't think anyone wants to be the reason that grandma remains in pain, clinging onto a decaying body, just because she is afraid it will be too difficult on everyone else when she is gone.

Make sure to point out to everyone this idea of "identifies", so that they see, acknowledge and become aware of the relationship they have had with the dying person and what identities and associations they both have played in each other's lives. Point out that these roles are currently insignificant and should not be constantly brought up and rubbed in the face of their dying loved one.

As far as the person who is dying, if needed, you can go over the fact that though they did have roles in this life which played a part in enhancing the lives of others, they now can let those go of these roles and move on to the next chapter. They have fulfilled their duties.

Talking about this at least brings it to their attention and acknowledges the idea of assumed identities. Often, this is enough to unstick their attention from all the ins and outs of what parts they played in this life.

11.

Everybody's Got Something to Hide

In the story, "A Christmas Carol" by Charles Dickens, a weird ghost visits Ebenezer Scrooge in the night. This ghost is actually Scrooge's previous business partner, Jacob Marley. Marley is a creepy, dead spirit now, and as he enters the space of the bedroom, you can hear the sound of clanking chains and heavy breathing.

Scrooge is terrified, and asks Marley why he is wrapped in chains. Marley explains to Scrooge that each link is forged from a sin he had committed in his lifetime. This implies that he is now trapped and burdened down by all these links (sins) from this chain in the afterlife.

Trapped and burdened by sins.

Absolution from a Catholic priest, as well in some other religions, is done to free someone from the pain and gripping effects caused by the guilt of acts a person committed which he or she now regrets. This is accomplished by granting absolute forgiveness. In this manner, those acts will hopefully no longer adversely affect the person. This tradition is seen to be a necessary action to a person's spiritual salvation.

Apparently, these types of secrets hinder us in life and in

death.

I have heard stories and seen examples of health improving only when the person was asked if they had any secrets to confess. People on their deathbed, being agitated and resentful up until the point when they finally disclosed what they had been ashamed of and felt remorse over, at which point they then became calm, loving, peaceful and could now let go.

There was a recent story where a 90-year-old man sent a check for $50.00 and a letter of apology to the Public Works department of a small town in Utah, because 75 years earlier, as a teenager, he had stolen a stop sign. He said he was "trying to make restitution for all the mistakes he's made in the past". [5]

It is amazing what we will put ourselves through and the self-imposed "punishments" we suffer, based on what we have done that we feel guilt over:

A fellow counselor, colleague of mine, told me he once had a client who divulged that he had been feeling horrible guilt for a long time due to something he'd done years ago that he had never told his wife about. Apparently, a few days before they got married, he'd slept with a prostitute the night of his bachelor party.

In one of the following sessions, he asked this counselor if he should tell his wife about it. The counselor told him that it was totally his decision. The client eventually concluded that he should confess to her, but also pleaded with this counselor to go to the house with him for support when he revealed this transgression.

When they both arrived at the house, the wife was cleaning up around the kitchen. The client informed her that he had something he needed to talk to her about. The conversation went something like this:

Him: *"Honey, I have something to tell you that I feel horrible about… And I think I should tell you because it's eating me up inside."*

Her: *"What are you talking about?"*

Him: *"Well… uhm… you see… before we got married, on my bachelor's night… uhm… we were all drinking a lot and… well, there was this girl there and… well… honey, I'm so sorry… I slept with her!"*

Her: *"Oh that? Yeah, I already knew about that. Lisa told me you guys had some strippers over there and there was sex and all that kinda stuff."*

Him: *"What?!? You knew about this? Are you kidding me? You've let me live in spiritual torment over these last 15 years of our marriage and you've never told me you already knew about it? How could you?!?"*

He was mad at her for not letting on that she knew about the bad thing that he did.

Go figure…

* * *

Another counselor friend of mine told me her parents had been in a bad car accident and had to be helicoptered to different hospitals. Her mother was in intensive care for 30 days and in a coma. She had many broken bones throughout her body and it was unclear if she would ever survive. The doctors operated on her for hours. After a few weeks she eventually came around and regained consciousness, but the doctors were still unsure if she was going to make it.

When she could talk, she became very bitter and started blaming her husband for her condition. She complained that it was his fault for the accident, and how bad he was, and she kept spewing all these criticisms of how he had ruined her life and everything connected with it. Her husband was in a similar physical condition in a nearby hospital trying to recover from the same accident. After a few days of trying to reassure her mother that she shouldn't be so bitter, and to let her husband "off the hook" etc., it became evident that reasoning or reassurance would not help pop her out of her bad attitude.

She finally asked her mother, "*Is there something you have done that daddy doesn't know about?*" After a few minutes of hemming and hawing, her mother calmed down and started explaining that when they were dating, many years ago, she started going out with another man who was very handsome, and she had never told her husband about that. She had been sitting on this secret for their whole marriage. Suddenly, she got quite tranquil, quit her complaining, and stopped blaming her husband for everything. Her physical condition immediately improved, she eventually was able to reunite with her husband, go through their physical therapy sessions and live out the remaining days of their lives together.

* * *

A client's story applying this step:

"We received news that my girlfriend's mother was not doing well at all and was dying from a type of cancer she had been fighting for some months.

The relationship between my girlfriend and her mom had been very tumultuous and strained for a long time, and there was ill will between them. Her mom had been using heavy drugs for many years and was always in and out of bad relationships. She had a history of struggling and my girlfriend was bitter about the whole thing.

When we arrived, my girlfriend's mom was in bed and very weak.

I decided to first try to establish some hope, by asking if she'd ever had an "out-of-body" experience. She said she had experienced that, though it was drug-induced. We then discussed the idea of the spirit as being separate from the body, which seemed to provide some comfort for her.

It became obvious to me that the best thing that could happen in these last days would be for my girlfriend and her mom to salvage their relationship as much as possible and experience some harmony at the end of her mother's life.

I decided the most expedient way to do this would see if I could do the step where I got her mom to tell her daughter whatever it was she felt she had to say or things she had done that she regretted.

When I brought up the idea of her telling her secrets to her daughter, she kept bouncing out of it all, saying stuff like, "Well, I just keep trying to...." or "I've always done my best..."

Nonsense stuff like that. I caught it and called her on it.

I said, "Listen, I noticed you do this thing, like where you start talking about stuff unrelated to what I ask you about. You seem to do it when you get close to talking about something more personal."

I explained how secrets could cut a person's willingness to communicate openly and actually make them make them pull back from life and relationships. I told her nothing she could ever say would ever influence my opinion of her.

Then I said, "You need to spill all of your secrets... the things you most wish you'd never done."

At which point she spilled and spilled and spilled. For a full 2 ½ hours.

During this period, of her divulging all her regretful acts, some of which were pretty degraded and hard to listen to, I had to referee my girlfriend from reacting too badly because she'd try to interject.

When the mom stalled, I'd coax her to keep the narrative going with prompters like, "What happened next?" kind of thing.

We let her continue until she felt relief.

She said she'd been holding onto these secrets her whole life and hadn't felt this good in 35 years.

She and her daughter hugged and cried, and for the next couple days were at each other's side in a harmonious and loving way until the mom passed away quietly and peacefully.

And my girlfriend's life goes on without any harmful hostility *toward the memory of her mother."*

* * *

Like the chains engulfing Jacob Marley, our sins seem to weigh us down and prevent us from moving on.

So, if needed, you may want to urge the person you are helping to allow you to relieve him or her of anything that they feel guilty about. If they are highly emotional over someone in their life, whether it is in a sad, regretful, angry or critical manner, they probably have done something they need to reveal before they can release and be free of all that harmful and trapped energy.

Guilt can bring about some powerful rationalizations and upsets, so be aware of the person in front of you and get them to divulge whatever is needed so they can feel relief and move on.

Remember, whatever they tell you, display absolutely no judgment. Do not ever violate their trust. Unless they say otherwise, let them know that what they disclose to you is under strict confidence and will go no further.

There is a lot of theory and information behind all this and how it works, but the previous stories illustrate what can happen when you help someone reveal those secrets that are "eating them up".

I realize that divulging secrets and confessing transgressions is usually a function left for priests and other religious personnel to perform, but like the examples above, sometimes the situation presents itself when your helping someone at the end of life.

Because you are there, you may need to assist them in this manner. Since you have been present, listening, giving guidance and showing compassion, you will be a safe outlet for those that really need someone to hear them.

Embrace it.

12.

I Hope I Die Before I Get Old

That's a line from a song called *"My Generation"*. It was recorded by a rock group called "The Who" in 1965, and was written by their guitarist, Pete Townshend.

He was 20 years old then. Today he is 73.

How about *"When I'm Sixty-Four"* written by Paul McCartney when he was about 15 years old. There's also the line from the 1966 Rolling Stones, Jagger-Richards song, *"Mother's Little Helper"*, with the line, *"What a drag it is getting old."* Mick and Keith were 23 when they recorded this.

When we say someone is getting old, exactly what is it that is aging or getting old? This has always fascinated me.

There are physicists who claim that the concept of Time is simply an illusion made up of human memories. Everything that has ever been and ever will be is happening right now. [6]

It's like when Yogi Berra was asked the question, "What time is it?", he replied, *"You mean now?"*

If you sit yourself down and begin remembering the details of specific times when you were young, it may eventually become evident, and you'll most likely figure out that *you* have not really changed very much at all.

Theoretically, as far as *you* are concerned, there is no "then". There is only "now".

You are who you are now, and you *were* who you are now, *then*.

Your elementary school looks different today, the house you grew up in has changed, and when you look in the mirror, your body has more sags, spots and wrinkles than it used to.

But *you* have remained a constant in each "now" of life.

It is easy to see change in the environment around us, but no one seems to acknowledge the fact that his or her body is part of that environment. Many believe they are their body. The body changes. Cells in the body change. Opinions change. The environment changes. But evidently, *you* really don't.

You have a body, just as you have a car and a house, an arm, a leg and a brain. But *you* are not inherently any of those solid things.

This concept that "you have always been pretty much the same you" is a workable model that seems to help orient the application of these steps when you are providing assistance to someone at the end of his or her life.

So, how does this apply to an aging body? It is sometimes hard for people to grasp that fact because our perception of ourselves often doesn't really want to acknowledge when our body actually is old, with all the problems and liabilities surrounding it.

When you're a little kid and you see grandma lying in a hospital bed, with all those tubes and pain and overwhelm, you might think to yourself, *"I'll never allow myself get to a point where that could happen to me"*.

But when your body matures to the age that your grandma was when you decided all this, you'll have a different perspective. You won't really think of it all ending because you, yourself, won't really consider you as "old" like your grandma appeared way back then. You can still see and think and enjoy certain things, so why consider finality to this life. It's not so bad.

And you can go on in this state of "not so bad" for many years.

I know it's sometimes hard to admit that the body is old. We have all heard people say things like, *"I know I'm old but I'm still young at heart"*. And it's true.

So, this brings us to the question: *"When is it appropriate to start end of life discussions?"*

In a book I mentioned earlier, *"Being Mortal"*, Doctor Atul Gawande details how he must deal with subjects like old age, disease, preservation of life, death and all the difficult decisions and opinions that surround us when that time arrives.

Here's the all too familiar scenario:

The husband's legs won't work anymore so he needs

a walker or has to be pushed in a wheelchair. No more stairs. His kidneys have failed so he'll need to be on dialysis machines 2-3 times a week. Someone must drive him there. He can't dress himself or handle the restroom alone. He starts getting dementia and forgets everyone who has been helping him all this time. He can't be home anymore, so where will he go and who is going to care for him there?

His life has been reduced to just "physically existing" and the lives of the loved ones close to him have evaporated into a tacitly, agreed-upon caretaker role.

I don't know the answer to all this, but I do know that there should be a conversation about the end of life details before it all turns for the worse. It's a "sensitive subject" with an unavoidable reality.

You wouldn't believe the percentages of those that claim to want to discuss their end of life details and those that actually do. 90% say it's an important conversation. Only 27% will have that discussion. [7]

Inheritances, wills, possessions, lawyers, do-not-resuscitate waivers, funeral arrangements etc., all should be figured out when everyone has their full faculties intact.

But studies show that most people won't go there.

The steps in this book were intended for those at the end of life, but I feel that maybe some of the information here could be applied in some fashion before someone is in their last few days.

It may be hard for family members to have these conversations with their parents. Maybe their parents would feel more comfortable talking with someone outside of the family.

You can encourage discussions about their beliefs, wishes, others that they have seen pass away, experiences dealing with older people etc., which may be a gentle approach to opening up a conversation around all this.

And what about you and your own life and death? Hopefully you will inform your loved ones of your wishes regarding what you want to happen at the end of your own life, so that everyone can carry on now without that "elephant in the room", wondering if they should bring it up or leave it alone as time goes on. What if your life was suddenly taken from you now by an accident or illness? Would your loved ones know what to do? Or would they be in a panic with all the decisions that comes when a death occurs?

It seems like the details of your death should be worked out when you're alive.

Don't put off taking care of the hard decisions and specific details regarding what you want to happen at the end of your own life. Inform your loved ones of your plans. Be open about it. Make those arrangements now, so that when it's your time, those you care about won't have the additional burden of having to figure out what your wishes might have been.

(I wonder if Pete Townsend still feels the same now as he did when he was 20. Hope not.)

13.

Human Touch

When you injure yourself, what is the first thing you do? You put your hand on the hurt body part, right?

Out of all the senses we as humans possess, touch is the most intimate. We can see things that are miles away. Our hearing extends a long way out from where our ears are located on our heads. Pleasant or not, we can smell all sorts of odors from a distance.

But touch is right here, right now. Touch means our skin is in direct contact with someone or something.

Even statements like, *"That song touched me."*, *"He is out of touch with reality."* and *"Please stay in touch."*, are all talking about connection and being connected.

Touching seems to be a common practice for a number of things. A kid hurts his knee. Mom gently touches the injured spot and he stops crying. The Christian practice of the "Laying of Hands" was associated with receiving the Holy Spirit. A doctor, placing his hands around the area with a, *"Does that hurt?"* means that the two of you are both engaged in an assessment of what may be wrong with your body and so re-establish your physical well-being.

I've learned and witnessed that fiddling gently with the toes of a newborn child can help them calm down after having just been delivered. Somehow the awareness that they are being connected with physically is an orientation and reassurance, after having been through an ordeal like childbirth.

A Speech Therapist I know told me that she went to the hospital to visit her father who had just undergone heart surgery. He was experiencing extreme pain due to the operation. She asked the doctor why he wasn't being given pain medication. The doctor pointed to the monitor that showed that his blood pressure was very low and because of this, taking pain medicine was too dangerous.

When the doctor left the room, she started placing her hand on various areas of her dad's body, ensuring he could feel her touch each time. As she continued in this manner, she noticed an increase in his blood pressure on the monitor. She continued this touching technique and watched the monitor to the point that her father's blood pressure now showed normal.

She called the doctor in and requested her dad now be given the pain meds. The doctor looked at the monitor and couldn't believe it. This simple technique of touching returned her dad's blood pressure to normal in a matter of minutes.

Hell, even puppies snuggle up to their mother for protection and a sense of security.

We instinctively do this when we are greeting someone. Shaking hands in a firm way shows acceptance of each other. Holding grandma's arm when she is bed-ridden helps the two of you connect. Hugging, stroking someone's hair, embracing, all these actions show that you care and therefore, have a healing quality.

I have listed this touching technique here to emphasize its workability in calming someone down who is in the process of his or her life coming to a close. Touching can also be used as a means of helping someone pull out of illnesses or injury. I have seen many examples of the power of touching and so wanted it included as a step to provide aid to someone.

Use it as needed to those you are helping.

14.

Stability

Have you ever had "the spins" when you lay down in a bed after you had too much alcohol to drink? You're lying there and things start to feel unstable, the room starts "moving", and you get nausea, along with a spinning sensation. The urban remedy has been to lie in your bed on your back, move a leg off the bed and place that foot squarely on the floor.

For some reason, being physically connected to a point of reference somehow gives a sort of stability to those situations.

A person, who is dying, often can be aided by drawing their attention to the physical environment around them. We have all seen this. We do it with little kids. The child is all upset and crying and you point to a flower in the grass and say something like, "*Look honey! Look at the beautiful flower.*" All of a sudden the crying stops and the kid calms down, while they investigate the flower in front of them.

This, or similar methods, can often pop a person out of an upset or confusion. These following techniques should be utilized as soon and as often as possible:

The dying person can often still see, feel, smell, hear and

touch the environment around them. Having them smell a flower, touch a bedspread, listen to a song, point to a picture in the room or visually locate the objects around them, can often be a stabilizing factor.

Showing them a photo album or drawings from their grandkids, and have them describe what they are seeing, can help bring their attention off their immediate situation. Anything that brings their attention outward to the environment is valid and stabilizing.

If they are unconscious or in some delirium, having them feel and touch the objects around them, by taking their hand and having them physically touch things in their reach, bed sheets, pillows, objects and body parts, can sometimes pull them out of it and restore their awareness.

Another way of helping is giving them something to do. Something as simple as, *"Please hand me that cup grandma"* will lift her spirits. *"Tell me what you think I should do about_____"* will put her in a better position because she will take to the role of helping.

Holding their hand or placing your hand on their shoulder when you speak, gives them more confidence by providing a physical connection to you.

Asking them to look at things in the room, until they seem calmer, is another stabilizing procedure.

Placing your palm on different areas of their body and asking if they can feel it provides an orientation to an often-overwhelming condition of being out-of-control.

Telling them to conceptually prevent their hands, feet, legs, arms, etc. from "leaving" diminishes a fear of departure because it is a reminder that they still can control something. This is accomplished with the simple directive, "Prevent your right foot from leaving. Prevent your left foot from leaving." and repeat on other body parts until the person seems better.

Having them describe objects near them, focuses their attention outwardly and can bring them into more "presence" than if you just talked to them.

If possible, wheeling them out of the room to an outdoor environment can do wonders for their outlook.

* * *

The point is, being on your "deathbed" can be an introverting and confusing time. Bringing someone's attention outward into the world to the things around them helps steady the confusion and provides more orientation and consciousness for them. Allowing the dying person to demonstrate ability, no matter how small, will help his or her emotional state of mind and outlook. Any of these stabilizing and orienting steps can really help in a big way.

15.

The Human Spirit

"Death comes to experience, not to you"

(Deepak Chopra)

Question: What future does someone have once his or her body has died?

Answer: No one knows.

Imagine, lying in a bed with people staring at you and treating the situation like this is the end of you... forever.

Allowing others to carry on around grandma, talking, implying or putting the idea out there that she is never going to exist, never, ever again, may be a bit upsetting to her, even if subconsciously.

Maybe it's true, but you don't have to rub it in her face. Keep your emotions positive and allow the person at the end of life to have some dignity and hope, or at least not continually being reminded of his or her own mortality.

Here is an approach:

There is a concept called the "Body-Mind-Spirit" model. It is well known. It is an idea that most people can accept to explain the whole of a person. They have a body, they use their mind to figure out solutions to living and they *are* the spirit (human soul) who oversees that organization called "Myself".

It is sometimes comforting to a person at the end of life to remind them of this idea, and that though it is true that their body will eventually perish, evidence shows that you, the spirit, will continue.

Just make sure you don't push this concept if it conflicts with something the person believes to be true. It's just a model that can be referred to offer hope.

Some functional definitions that I came up with:

The Body – The physical manifestation of a person. A vessel the person uses to live a life on planet earth. A body without an active and aware spirit would probably be, more or less, like a zombie walking around looking for food. The average lifespan of a human body at this writing is 79 years. The brain is physical and is part of the body. The brain and the body will die.

The Mind – The operation and mechanism the spirit uses and deploys to forward the identities he or she has assumed and taken on in this life. It is unknown if the mind perishes fully or is possibly retained to some degree by the spirit.

The Spirit – The Human Soul. Consciousness. Life Force. The Being. *You*. The spirit uses the mind and exists in and around the body but is neither the body nor the mind. It is not physical. It is basically indefinable in physical terms. The spirit is the "constant" throughout your life. If you recall being very young and what you were doing at the time, you may realize that *you*, at this moment, and *you* back at that earlier moment, are pretty much the same *you,* even though your body looks totally different now and you may have different opinions from when you were younger.

At death, *you,* the spirit, apparently separate from the body.

* * *

There has been the observation that the body loses 21 grams of weight at body death. That's the weight of a hummingbird or a small candy bar. [8]

It is my opinion that this could be the soul departing the body, and the weight is possibly the "mental machinery" and/or memory banks contained in the mind.

Where the spirit goes or what happens after body death is based on the belief and faith of that individual.

And while we are on the subject, how did these bodies we inhabit come about in the first place? Are we from clay, apes or aliens?

Since the beginning of time, everyone is always asking the question, *"Where do we come from?",* but neither religion nor science have provided an answer that the world can agree on. In other words, when and how did our human bodies originate.

Genesis, the first book in the Bible, states, *"...the Lord God sent man out of the garden of Eden to till the ground from which he was taken.* (Genesis 3:23). Apparently, Adam (man) was made from clay and then, from his rib, Eve (woman) was created.

The Theory of Evolution, as outlined by Charles Darwin, suggests that a species undergoes continuous changes that are manifested over generations, and the main driving force that brought about these changes was the organism's instinct to survive. Nature automatically selects the useful traits and gets rid of those that are less important or necessary. This process apparently led to the emergence of *Homo sapiens,* from a distinct species of the hominid family, the great apes.

As detailed in the book, "*The 12th Planet*" by Zecharia Sitchin, the earliest known civilization on earth, Sumer, engraved characters on tablets 4500 years before Christ. Those tablets have now been translated. These writings make claims that the first human beings on earth were genetically engineered from the cells and DNA of an advanced alien race called, "The Anunnaki", which were then combined with the DNA from a bipedal, tool-using, large-brained primate (ape-like) from this planet. The stories in Genesis are said to have originated from these ancient claims, using names like, "Eden", "Adam" and "Eve", which were actually altered words and concepts from this alien race.

When it comes to body death, we may want to investigate somewhat how these bodies came about in the first place. Right now, it's an open market; so don't judge anyone's opinion as wrong.

Remember, the Body-Mind-Spirit concept is just a model. A theory. A way to explain the unexplainable. Science has yet to accurately define the human spirit and so we have faith, religion and belief to give different explanations and hope.

The point is, if applicable, provide hope to the dying that they are not actually going to perish. It's not your place to tell them what to believe but I have had some success in reminding the person that, yes, their body is going to die but they are *not it*. They are not their body.

There are many that believe they will keep going, if not as a consciousness, at least the effects that they have created on others and the fact that their contributions will carry on long after they have departed. Like the story illustrated in the movie, "It's a Wonderful Life", we have all touched the lives of others and that influence carries on long after we have passed away.

Letting go of a dying body is more difficult if a person feels it will be the complete end of everything. The idea that he or she will be part of a continuation of life can often assuage fears and make it easier to let go and move on.

16.

List Out Their Concerns or What They Have Attention On

This step has you ask the dying person if there is anything that he or she is worried about or is causing distress, and then let them know you'll get it addressed.

This is another step to help get their attention freed up so that they don't have these types of concerns, fears and doubts haunting them during the final days of this life.

I have seen people having attention on things like, *"Tell my daughter that the circuit breaker at the house will trip if the heater and vacuum cleaner on going at the same time"*. Or, *"My husband doesn't know how to pay the bills. Could you please see that he learns?"*

I mean, look at your own life. If you had to suddenly move to another part of the world, and you had to leave now, what would you have your attention on that you'd want taken care of? It's probably unfinished situations or projects. We don't ever look at the fact that these things tie up our thoughts and how great we feel when we finally get rid of that stack of junk in the garage or fix that thing or call that person or send that thank you card we've been meaning to get to.

People feel relieved when they know things are getting completed. Those at the end of life can be greatly helped by finding out what it is that they're concerned about and letting them know you're on it.

17.

List Out What They Want to Say

People often put-off saying things until it's too late.

How about that really great college professor? Have you ever contacted him and told him how much you learned in his class? How about the person who mentored you at the start of your career? Did you ever thank them for ensuring you really got what was going on? How about your parents for raising you? Your kids for making a good life for themselves? Your friend for always being there? Your wife or husband for the life they have shared with you?

After high school, I worked for a small construction company. My boss was a hard-ass and yelled at me all the time. He would constantly push me to do more, learn faster, keep things organized, find something to do to improve the jobsite, master the tools I was using and develop the skills necessary toward the basics of construction and building houses. At the time, I didn't realize what effect this mentoring (and berating!) would have on me. I just thought he was being mean.

I eventually went into a career of coaching and counseling, but I always retained my ability as a carpenter.

Thirty years later, with the help of a friend of mine, we

built an addition to my house that included a library, great room, bathroom and huge kitchen. About half way into the project, I was looking around at the work we'd done and realized that it was my old boss who had given me the ability to create these extra rooms to expand and improve my home.

Through an old friend from my hometown, I found his phone number and called him. He answered. I explained to him that I was putting an addition on my house and I wanted him to know how appreciative I was for his incredible instruction all those years ago. I let him know that what he taught me helped me not only as a carpenter, but in everything I have done in my life.

I really wanted to let him know that his instruction and guidance gave me lasting abilities that I could never have obtained on my own.

This tough-guy-boss started crying for being acknowledged in this way.

I am so glad I gave him that message before he died, where I'd never again get the chance.

Finding out what messages someone at the end of life wants relayed, is a comforting step for him or her. The relief they can experience knowing that their unspoken communications will be delivered, can help put them in a very calm state of mind and provide them a closure to those people and chapters of their life.

Whatever way you want to word it is up to you:

"Are there any messages you'd like me to deliver to anyone?"

"Is there anybody you'd like me to get ahold of and tell them something you'd like them to know?

"Let me know any people you'd like me deliver a message to and tell me what you'd like to say to each of them."

If there is someone special they want to get a message to, and you can arrange for that person to be present, in person, all the better.

18.

Requests

I thought I should mention something that I have seen around this area of those at the end of life or even some with disabilities. It has to do with quality of life versus just keeping a body alive.

Sometimes you may be confronted with requests that go against rules or advices from a medical professional or family member. The person asks for something that the doctor said they shouldn't have. This sometimes does create a dilemma. I guess you'll have to decide, based on the greater good, on how to approach it:

* * *

A medical director I know worked in a hospital caring for those that were heavily disabled. One man had what's called "Locked-in Syndrome". He was in a permanent state where he couldn't move anything except his eyes, he couldn't swallow, he couldn't walk, and he could no longer move his arms. They had to use an Augmentative Communication System, where the healthcare staff used an alphabet board, pointing to the individual letters so he could then blink on the correct one, and therefore spell the word he wanted to say.

One day he spelled the word "hamburger". He wanted a hamburger. He pleaded day after day to allow him this one wish. He couldn't swallow, so based on the perspective of the medical profession, to grant this request was out-of-the-question. The liability and risks were too high.

However, this medical director pushed until his request was finally approved through an Ethics Committee. It took a long time. She had to get all these release papers "signed" by the patient saying that the hospital could not be held responsible for any bad outcome that may occur from him "eating" a hamburger. Because he had no ability to chew or swallow, there was a danger of something getting lodged in his esophagus with no means of moving it through, and the patient then choking to death.

After all the waivers were signed, the day finally came when this guy could get his hamburger.

She said she got the burger and brought it to his room. He was visibly excited. She cut a piece of the burger, bun and all, and gently placed it on his tongue. She waited. After a minute or so she removed the hamburger from the patient's mouth and noticed he had tears in his eyes.

Tears of happiness.

What would you have done? Apathetically accept a general rule and protocol or take the necessary steps required to provide a sense of dignity and self-determinism to someone who had none?

* * *

There was another instance where a father was at the end of life in the hospital with a respiratory condition. His son and daughter-in-law were visiting. He told them he'd like a cup of coffee but they explained that the doctors said caffeine was not good for him, so "no" on the coffee.

They continued their visit but eventually told their dad they'd return later that evening after they went home for dinner. An hour after they left the hospital room, he died.

And he never got that last cup of coffee.

* * *

When you are helping others there will be always be situations and questions that will present themselves. She wants you to wheel her outside, so she can have a cigarette. He wants to leave the hospital and go home now, no matter what the outcome. Do we do further medical procedures or provide hospice? These are not easy decisions to make.

Advanced Medical Directives can and should be utilized before things turn for the worse, so that specific requests and special needs can be communicated as needed.

If confronted with a request that seems go against what is allowed by the doctor, talk to the staff and find out the reality of what it may take to being able to grant that request. It might take some thought and effort to pull it off, but at least you'll have the two examples above as something to contemplate when the dying person's wishes conflict with medical advices.

19.

Leave the Room

Do you like people watching you go to the bathroom? How about crowds staring at you while you deliver a baby? Hell, I don't like it when I get hurt or sprain an ankle and someone rushes over starts in on me, *"Are you okay? What happened? Are you hurt? Can you walk?"* I'd much rather just be with myself to deal with what I need to deal with until the pain and confusion has diminished. I don't want to be distracted by a bunch of frantic communication from others.

Maybe the dying person doesn't want you in the room staring at them when they are ready to go.

I've seen this in many cases. Nurses and hospice personnel have verified it. You'll have people in the vicinity of the hospital bed all day and night, hovering around the dying person, crying, solemn, pleading etc., and as soon as everyone leaves for dinner or maybe a shower (having been up all night), that's when the dying dies.

With no one around watching.

I have to think there is something to this. I imagine actually dying, with all the physical shut down and separation from the body, takes a bit of concentration. Having your attention on a room full of people, while at the same time "letting go", may create a more confusing, difficult and a less peaceful process.

Periodically leave the room and ensure everyone else does the same.

20.

These Are Days You'll Remember

Joke:

Wife: *"What did the doctor say?"*

Husband: *"He told me, based on my condition, I've only got a few more hours to live."*

Wife: *"That's horrible! What should we do?"*

Husband: *"Well, I thought maybe we could have a nice dinner with wine, then sit by the fire with some brandy and talk about our life together and then I just want to make love with you all throughout the night."*

Wife: *"Oh. Ah… yeah… well… I don't know… uhm… see, actually, I've gotta get up in the morning."*

* * *

In reality, the people around the deceased are going to continue living. There will be loss but realize that there is loss all throughout life.

Dropping the 5-year-old off at his or her first day of school is totally traumatic for some mothers. But soon, that emotion dissipates and life resumes. Apparently it is set up that way.

Often, our lives have been extremely interrupted and taxed due to the care and concern we have extended to our loved one over the days, months and sometimes years of disability. When it is all over, it is mainly what happens in the end that we will remember.

If you were having a blast at a family reunion all day but in the early evening one of your uncles got too drunk, started a fight with another guest where things got broken, your uncle cut his forehead on the corner of a table, the police had to be called, and your grandma got all upset because the whole party had to be disbanded, what image would remain in your mind years after that reunion?

If you went to a great rock concert for a couple hours but on your way home, you got into a car accident and your boyfriend had to get stitches in the hospital, and then two years later, someone asked you how that concert was, what would be your remembrance of that night?

If you were climbing a mountain, enduring hardship, starvation and lack of sleep, but still made it to the peak and achieved your goal, would that climb end up being a good memory or a bad memory?

If the pregnancy was taxing, the labor exhausting and the childbirth extremely painful, yet in the end, you're able to hold your brand-new, healthy baby daughter in your arms, was all worth it? Is that a good memory?

It has been observed that it is the end of an event or situation that seems to be the thing we remember most. If the ending is good or fulfilling, all the oppressive obstacles, physical pain, emotional stress and spiritual suffering you had to go through are overlooked and the overall memory of the whole thing will be predominantly good. If the end of an event turns out bad or traumatic, that perception will be at the forefront in our mind as far as what we remember about it. We've all heard statements like, *"Oh, that movie was okay, but the ending sucked. I wouldn't even bother to see it if I were you."*

This is another reason why it is important to help make the last days of someone's life as peaceful and painless as possible, not only for the dying person but for the people who are there witnessing it all. The end of someone's life is what will be prominent in the minds of those that live on.

Another aspect to this is the fact that there will be people around the dying person who won't know what they should do or say. They will be at a loss, and your direction can help them. Something as simple as, *"Go in the room, hold your grandma's hand, remind her of the times you spent together and thank her for all she's done for you"*. That simple directive can really help say goodbye in a meaningful way and close out that chapter of life for everyone involved. The memory of that final event will much better that way.

Remember, you now can help provide the best possible conclusion to a person's life and the memories in the lives of his or her loved ones.

21.

Contradictions

"He who would do good to another must do it in minute (tiny, exact) particulars. General "Good" is the plea of the scoundrel, hypocrite, and flatterer, for Art and Science cannot exist but in minutely organized particulars."

(William Blake)

When I was proofreading through the various pages of this book, trying to ensure is reads well and makes sense; I realized that there might be parts and steps that seem like they contradict each other.

Sorry, but life is pretty much filled with contradictions:

"I love my teenager, but she drives me crazy."

"I hate my job, but I like the money."

"My husband is really smart, but he spaces out too much."

Apparently, this subject matter is no exception, in that some of the advice written here may seem to say one thing and then later imply the opposite.

People are *individuals*. You'll never be able to do a blanket, general, overall action, because each person requires a personal touch. That's why the guideline, *"Help the person in front of you"* is so powerful. What is good for one person may be irrelevant to the next.

These steps must be intelligently applied to the person you're helping and based on his or her particular needs and hopes. Assess what you think will be the most logical actions to take, put them in a sensible sequence, and go ahead and start helping, even if it seems to contradict something.

Listening, not violating what that person believes, and genuinely caring for them, will take you through the process.

You may need to leave alone any mention of the idea of the human spirit. You may not be able to have any kind of communication other than touching them with a reassuring hand. They might not need much assistance at all, other than you just being there and acknowledging their attitude, which can help them more than anything else you thought you were going to provide them.

Trust yourself and you'll do great with however you decide to move forward with your support.

22.

The Letter

Let's say your name is Jamie.

One day, when your mail arrives there is a package. You open it, and it's a book. The title of the book says, "*Letters to Jamie*", with a picture of you on the cover.

You start flipping through and see that every page is a letter to you from someone you have known. Siblings, cousins, previous schoolmates, past kids from your neighborhood, people you've worked with, college friends, and even some people you haven't thought of in years.

Each letter talks about how much you have helped them, fun times you had together, hilarious moments you've shared, in what ways you've enhanced their life and basically how awesome and appreciated you are.

I bet you would read every page of that book.

These letters are examples of the types of commentaries you most often hear at memorials regarding the deceased. But why do we wait until someone has died before we let them know how great they are?

People are usually at a loss as to what to do when someone is dying. As the person taking control in this type of circumstance, you will be inundated with people asking and saying things like:

"How can I help?" "Can I do anything?" "I am so sorry..."

Those who are helping a dying person must also deal with the living. People will be emailing you, calling you, texting you and writing to you.

How do you address all of these people who are concerned?

One of the biggest regrets people have after someone has died is what they were *not* able to say to them. What they will never again have the chance to communicate to them, now that they are gone.

This seems to be one of the heaviest losses for most people.

"I'll never get to tell her how much she meant to me."

"I wanted to tell him I love him and now I'll never be able to."

"I wanted to thank her for helping me that one time and now I can't."

I have found that there will be people from all over the country that are friends and family who will be affected by this situation.

Because of this fact, you should instruct everyone who has a connection to the person who is dying, to write a one-page email letter, describing everything they want to say, and tell them you'll put it in a book so you can read it to their loved one.

Create a group email and send them something along the following:

"Dear friends and family of [dying person's first name] ,

Many of you have written and called me asking how you can help. Here's how:

Each of you email me a one-page letter to [dying person's first name].

Include everything you want (him/her) to know; good times you had together, how (he/she) helped influence your life, thank (him/her) for whatever you want, and let (him/her) know any details as to how special (he/she) is to you.

Try to keep your personal feelings of loss out of the letter as much as possible. [Dying person's name] *can't do anything about your upset. (He/she) has enough to deal with right now.*

I will create a book out of all these letters and read them to [dying person's name] *every chance I can.* [He/she] *will love to hear from you and this book will help lift (his/her) spirits.*

The book will be called "Letters to [dying person's name]*". I'll make sure you can get a copy of it.*

Do not wait. Write that email and send it to me now."

* * *

When this has been done, it has helped everyone involved.

The person on their deathbed really enjoyed hearing how they had influenced and positively affected the lives of their loved ones and friends everywhere.

All the people who wrote letters were able to finalize things by expressing everything they wanted to say and were able to have a sort of closure on that chapter of their lives.

The book is then made available at the memorial or funeral for all to take home and read through. Copies can also be mailed to those who couldn't make it to the bedside or funeral.

Any office supply store can put together a book of these letters once you have received the emails from everyone.

Like I've mentioned, the ending part of situations or events in our lives are what people remember most, so the implementation of this book of letters helps the dying before they pass as well as providing a sense of closure for the living around them.

23.

This May Be The Last Time

The 10-year-old is in heavy grief and loss over the fact that she knows her grandpa is dying. He and her have had a very close relationship and her heart is breaking. What should you do?

In the 1930's movie, "Angels with Dirty Faces", the kids in the neighborhood worship the local mob criminal who defies everything. He steals, he murders, he's violent, he's tough, has lots of money and appears to be "above it all", basically a type of urban hero to a poor, underprivileged 14-year old.

Well, at the end of the movie he gets caught and is sentenced to death by electrocution. A local priest pleads with this criminal to not allow his final message to these kids the perception that he is some courageous role model. The clergyman urges him to break the fantasy that the criminal life is one to aspire to.

In the last scene, you wonder what this mobster will do, when suddenly, as he's getting put into the electric chair, you hear him screaming and crying, *"No, no… please don't kill me! I don't want to die. I am scared, I'm sorry… please, please let me live!"*

When the story comes out in the newspaper the next day, the kids are all upset and in disbelief that their hero is actually a coward. But of course, it now gives them a chance to strive for something better than a life of crime.

The last words of the dying can help the living, especially the younger ones.

There may be those around the scene that really need some direction or reassurance from the person at the end of life. If possible, persuade the person who is dying to deliver to his or her loved ones whatever communications are needed to accomplish that reassurance.

In the example of the grandfather to his 10-year-old granddaughter, it could be something like this:

"Honey, I'll always love you. You know that. You need to be who you are and not change yourself to please others. Create your life in the way that you know is best for you. I'm forever proud of you. Now go out into the waiting room and give your mom a hug. She needs one."

That little girl will never forget her grandpa's last words to her.

Section Four

STRANGE MAGIC

If the daughter, whose mother just passed away three days ago, calls you up and tells you how her "mom" came to her last night at 3 in the morning, and starts explaining about the telepathic conversation they had, what are you going to say?

24.

Paranormal Encounters

Paranormal: *"Denoting events or phenomena such as telekinesis or clairvoyance that are beyond the scope of normal scientific understanding"*.

There are too many stories, assertions and crazy-weird instances that I have actually seen, experienced or been described to by others, that this subject of paranormal and inexplicable types of phenomena has to be included in this book.

This is because you may be faced with these types of things when you're helping someone at the end of life or in dealing with their families. I have.

I am making no claims about what you'll read here. It's only what I have experienced and what certain individuals have said to me regarding what they themselves have observed and been subjected to.

(Note: I don't consider these people to be crazy or delusional. The individuals with the stories you will be reading here, are all, relatively conservative, normal people.)

Science doesn't offer much of anything on these subjects, so we are left with the experiences of the people who have witnessed events that seemed out-of-the-ordinary and incomprehensible.

I am including each of the categories in this section because of the subject matter and observations that have been brought up by either my clients or those they were helping. I wanted you to be aware of what others have talked about, so you won't get thrown off if you are confronted with similar instances.

Like I keep repeating, it isn't your place to tell anyone what to think or believe. None of that matters. You are there to give direction and listen. If you hear something you don't agree with or seems unreal, so what? Maybe you need to listen to it all the way through. You might learn something.

Remember, science can't explain this stuff.

You are there to comfort and be effective, not to judge.

Off we go into the wild blue yonder...

25.

Out-of-Body Experiences

This one is quite prevalent as a concept, but no one seems to ever take it to its next logical conclusion.

I asked the following question in the first episode of the podcast series, "It's the Question":

"Have you ever been outside of your body?"

We got lots of answers. Believe me.

Many people have claimed to have been out of their bodies at one or more points in their life. Some had instances that were induced by drugs, some had bad accidents and felt forced out and watched the scene from an exterior viewpoint, some had been in operations and surgeries and looked down on the whole thing from eight feet above it. Others claimed to have been in a meditative state or a counseling session and felt themselves moving out of their physical body in a very controlled and pleasurable way.

Even people that answered "no" to that question, saying they had not been out of their body, gave explanations as to why they thought it had not occurred. They never questioned the possibility of it. They just felt that the types of circumstances that would cause an out-of-body experience had never happened to them. Incredibly, the people answering "no" were still not denying the fact that it could happen.

No one responded with, "*What are you talking about?*" or asked to clarify that concept. Not one person denied the possibility of that type of phenomena, even if it had never happened to them.

This fact is just amazing to me.

And guess what? No one ever seems to put together this one simple, obvious aspect of out-of-body experiences:

If you can leave the body at any point in your life, wouldn't that mean *you* are not your body? If you have left or gotten out of something, you are other than the thing you claim to have gotten out of. Right?

There's another facet to this; many people that answered "yes", and described a time they had been out of their body, mentioned that they could see the room from the ceiling or they were above the building or neighborhoods and were able to see everything from that exterior vantage point.

I remember hearing a talk from a doctor, who told the story of a girl who had been blind since birth, waking up after having been in a lengthy operation, explaining everything she was able "see" while outside of her body during the procedure. She described perfectly what had visually gone on in that room when she was unconscious. She said it was a 360-degree visual perception, and she was completely astounded about all this, having never before seen anything in her entire life.

What these people have all described is, *seeing without using their body's eyes.*

Wow! How does that work?

Think about it, if you can be outside of your own head, brain, kidneys, legs, fingernails and every other body part, what are *you* then? If you can all of a sudden become exterior to your body and see the room and the environment without the body's eyes, how far up and out could you theoretically go?

If you can be aware of the scene in front of you, from a viewpoint outside of your physical body, and you can retain that experience as a memory, then what does the brain have to do with memory and what does the body have to do with what we are sensing?

Makes one think, doesn't it?

In his best selling book *"Proof of Heaven"*, Eben Alexander M.D. describes what occurred to him in a near death experience. Because of his profession, his beliefs about our existence as humans had been merely physical. Spiritual and religious ideas were just that, ideas with no validity. This all changed however, when he got extremely ill and went into a coma for several days. No one thought he would make it. He miraculously regained consciousness and described what he had experienced during the time he was basically thought to be dead. His statement was along the lines of, *"We've had it all wrong. We are not physical. We are consciousness"*.

Though I could tell a multitude of stories and examples of people claiming to have had an out of body experience, the following is interesting to me because of its context to the subject matter of this book:

A client once told me about a time it was near the end of a yoga exercise class he was participating in. The instructor had the class wind down by having them get into a certain relaxed body position, close their eyes and go into a mental, peaceful silence for a short period of time.

All of a sudden the instructor gave the directive, "*Okay, now step out of your body.*"

My client said he immediately felt himself move up and out of his physical body, through the ceiling and above the building's structure, looking down from a viewpoint a couple hundred feet above the roof. He said he could see the roof of the building and the entire city from this vantage point.

He said it was a bit scary, yet exhilarating.

After he settled back in and composed himself, after this new enlightening experience, people were leaving the class and he witnessed a woman berating the man in charge of the yoga session. She was visibly upset.

She told the instructor she didn't appreciate him giving the type of direction that conflicted with her Christian beliefs. Apparently, this new out-of-body experience startled her, and this reality somehow was a violation of the way she believed things were supposed to be, according to her faith.

This is one of these contradictions I mentioned earlier in the book. Even if someone is exposed to "evidence" that conflicts with what they believe in, it doesn't mean it will alter or stop them from their faith.

Faith and belief are personal to each person, so tread lightly when entering this area with someone at the end of life and the friends and family around them.

As previously stated, the Body-Mind-Spirit model is something to consider regarding death of the body. If we can have out-of-body experiences when the body is alive, then possibly we will still exist when the body perishes.

It seems like maybe this would be a good conversation to have with someone at the end of life. Ask them if they have ever had an out-of-body experience. If they answer "yes", point out that it is possible, that they are not their body and that they might continue to exist no matter what the condition of their physical body is in.

A client of mine did this with his dying mother-in-law and it worked well because it gave her some hope. Try it if it seems applicable.

26.

Telepathy, Clairvoyance and Intuition

Joke:

Betty and Mabel had been friends for years but were now very old. They made an agreement with each other that the first one of them to pass away had to "come back" and let the other know what it's like in Heaven.

Sure enough, Betty died.

A month later, during the middle of the night, Mabel woke up to a whispering voice. *"Mabel, Mabel. It's me…"*

Mabel sat up and said out loud, *"Oh my gosh, you've come back! This is amazing. Tell me Betty, what is it like?"*

Betty's spirit replied, *"Well Mabel. It's not what we thought. We eat a lot of vegetables and we have lots of sex."*

Mabel responded, *"Really? Is that true? That's what it's like in Heaven?"*

Betty explained, *"Oh no Mabel, I'm not in Heaven. I'm a rabbit in Wisconsin."*

* * *

Have you ever heard the phone ring and just knew who it

was before even looking? Have you ever called someone, and they say, "*Wow! I was just thinking about you?* Have you ever just "known" something was wrong with a loved one and it turned out to be true? Have you ever been so in tune with another person that you both knew the concepts you were each thinking about without having to speak?

Telepathy or clairvoyance is another one of those things that everyone is aware of, but we don't really go much deeper into questioning how it can possibly be.

I've included this section because you may be confronted with this type of thing in some capacity from others around the scene you'll be in.

A few examples:

A client of mine was administering some of the steps included in this book with his father, who was on his deathbed in a hospice setting.

He let his dad know that it was possible that our true nature is spiritual and that there is a chance that he will continue after his body has stopped working. He also said, "*Dad, anytime you want to let go of your body, it's okay. And if you want to communicate with me afterwards, I will be able to "hear" you.*"

They spent some more quality time together that evening but eventually my client said "good night" and left for the long drive back to the house where the rest of the family was staying.

During the drive home, all of a sudden, he got a strong communication from his dad. It was very vivid and pervaded the entire space, in and around the car. He said this communication was confused and frantic as to what was happening. He said it was obvious that his dad had passed away, departed his body and was now at a loss as to what he should do.

Without the use of ears or vocal cords, my client telepathically acknowledged and comforted his father, letting him know that his body had just died but he was still himself and that together they could eventually figure out what to do next.

Suddenly, the space got calm, his dad (spirit) thanked him and that was it.

When my client arrived back at the house, the whole family came out to the driveway crying. They obviously had received a phone call from the hospital. When they all started to inform my client of the news they had just received, he quietly said, "*It's okay. I already know. Dad's gone.*"

* * *

Another client had a "feeling" there was something wrong with her father around 2:00 P.M. She was in Chicago and he was in Tennessee, 500 miles away.

Later that evening she got a call from her sister, telling her that her dad had fallen into the water from a small fishing boat, had a heart attack, and died at 2:00 P.M. earlier that day.

* * *

Another client told me her brother had been in the

hospital for some weeks with a terminal condition. She lives in California and her brother was in a hospital in North Carolina. She was making plans for another trip to go and see him.

We went over some of the steps in this book so she could provide some comfort and reassurance for him, as well as the other family members who would be there.

A few days before her scheduled flight, she said she got an awareness or intuition that she should go *now*.

She paid the extra money to change her ticket and took the next immediate flight out of California, which was a red eye. She arrived in North Carolina early that next morning.

When she got to the hospital, there were a bunch of family members there around the bed. Her brother was on morphine, in and out of consciousness. She touched him, told him she was there, that she loved him, thanked him for all he'd done for everyone, reassured him that everything was taken care of, his sons were going to be looked after and they were fine, and at any point he wanted to let go of his body, it was totally okay for him to do so. The rest of the room gasped at this, but she reassured her brother that it was his decision.

All of a sudden, he opened his eyes, sat up, looked around the room at everyone, and then fell back into his sleep.

She told him she was going to check into her hotel, get cleaned up, and would be back shortly. She got everyone else out of the room too.

When she got to the parking lot, on the way to her rental car, she got a call from the hospital saying she needed to come back now.

When she returned, she was told her brother had passed away a few minutes after everyone left the room.

She was so grateful that she had followed her perception to make that trip when she did. Otherwise she would have never gotten to help her brother through that process, tell him that she loved him, and had that last chance to say goodbye.

* * *

Another example of a type of telepathy (or something); a client told me her best friend died and she was so upset that she went to a psychic to try and get some answers. She told me what happened in that session:

Psychic: "*Someone very close to you has passed away. I get an "R"... Ra... Raquel... no, Rachel.* (It was Rachel)

Okay, now I'm picking up on something, something to do with bikes... and another woman... bikes... and I'm getting the name, Debbie".

All of a sudden my client said she started crying. She told the psychic that yes, her and Rachel would work out at the local health club every week, and together they would take a spin class with those exercise bikes. The instructor's name is Debbie. She couldn't believe the psychic could pick up on this.

Psychic: "*Yes, and Rachel wants you to know that she's happy that she no longer has to worry about losing weight.* (Totally

Rachel's humor). *And she also wants you to know that when you are talking to her in your car, she hears you, and you really are connecting with her, so don't discount it."*

My client had told me she would talk to her deceased friend out loud when she was driving. She said it was comforting and was amazed that the psychic was aware of all of this.

The session continued, and the psychic was able to relay a few more spot-on details regarding my client's friend and their relationship.

* * *

Just know that this telepathic and clairvoyant type of activity may be something that you will either experience or hear about from others.

Don't say I didn't tell you.

27.

We Have All Been Here Before

Past lives are well-known phenomena. Many books have been written on the subject. There are videos that have people explaining their experiences with past lives. You can google the subject and read many stories about it.

There are parents who have kids who have given names and information about their past identity, down to most detailed detail, and which could have never been told to them by anyone this lifetime.

Again, let's take this to the next logical conclusion. If it is possible that we have had prior lives and identities, wouldn't it also be possible that we may live again after this lifetime?

Below are a few examples and stories of what I have been told by clients I have known:

One woman from New Zealand was using the steps of this program to assist her dying mother there. She explained to her mom that it may be possible that we are spiritual beings and that we don't die, and if that is the case, we all have had past lives and will probably have future lives as well. Her mother replied, *"Well honey, I have always known that I've lived before. I just didn't realize it went by so quickly."*

Another woman, we'll call her Stacey, told me she had a long-time male friend who she grew up with in their neighborhood. We'll call him Kyle. Over the years, Kyle used to randomly just show up at Stacey's home, school or place of work and greet her with, *"Hey babe... how's it goin'?"*

At some point later, when Kyle was working with a construction company, there was a bad accident where a wall caved in on him and a few others, which killed them all.

Sometime after that, when Stacey was pregnant, she was asleep one night, when all of a sudden she was awoken because she felt some sort of obvious presence from this Kyle soul. He telepathically asked if it would be okay to be in her family, indicating he wanted to become the baby she was to deliver in a few months.

She said it was a very vivid and genuine communication.

A few months after that, the baby was born. A girl. One day when Stacey's little girl was three years old, and after a bath, she got out of the bathtub and said to her mother, *"Hey babe... I'm Kyle."*

* * *

Another client told me that one day, her 3-year-old little boy kind of snarled at her to, *"Get along Missy"*. The only person who had ever called her that or uttered that phrase was her father who had long since been dead, way before her son was born.

* * *

There was a client who told me one day when he was a little boy, he snuck up into his grandma's attic, exploring around, and he found a bunch of oil paintings under some tarps. He looked at these paintings and just knew he had painted them. He recognized every one of them, all the details of how he'd painted them and all the themes behind each one. He ran downstairs and asked his grandmother, *"Grandma, who painted all those pictures in the attic?"* She said, *"Oh yes... those were painted by your grandfather, years ago. And you know, you are so much like him!"*

His grandfather had died years before my client was ever born.

* * *

Another client, we'll call her Sandy, told me that when she was nine months pregnant with her second child, she got a phone call from a woman who introduced herself and explained that she had advanced cancer and was dying. The woman told Sandy that she had been referred to her, knew she was pregnant and asked if it would be okay to become part of Sandy's family, indicating she wanted to "be the baby" about to be delivered.

This woman explained that she had heard that Sandy's husband was a musician and that she herself was an artist, ran a school in Los Angeles and thought that it would be a good fit.

Sandy was kind of weirded-out by the call but half-heartedly replied, "Yeah... okay, I guess so.

The woman said, *"Great! I'm sending you a check for the baby's savings account* (which she did), *I have to turn over the school to someone who I am now training and then finalize a few other things. I'll be in touch."*

When Sandy was near the end of the 9th month, the woman called again. She said, *"Okay. I have wrapped everything up. I've turned over the school, trained my replacement there, and everything is now all set to go."*

That night the old woman passed away and the next morning Sandy delivered a baby girl.

About 4 years later, Sandy was in Los Angeles on a business trip, and took her daughter along with her. She decided to visit that school the woman said she had owned.

They entered the school together, and as they were walking down the hallway, her daughter was looking all around and then remarked, *"Mmm… they painted the place."*

* * *

The whole concept of Buddhism is to attain a state of enlightenment where you end the cycle of birth/death, birth/death, birth/death. The movie and book, "What Dreams May Come", details the act of dying and then being reborn into a new identity. "Heaven Can Wait" is the story of a man who died, did not agree with going to heaven right now, returned to earth, and started a new life in another body.

I know these movies are fiction, but why are these stories so compelling and why are there so many of them.

Again, referencing these stories and concepts can help soften the fear of becoming "nothing" at death, and give some hope, which may help when it is time to let go.

28.

When Does the Soul Enter Body?

Different religions and philosophies have divergent ideas as to when the soul enters and joins a human body. It is sometimes called "Ensoulment". Some feel the soul is created as the child develops while others who believe in reincarnation believe the soul is a separate entity and exists prior to conception.

Christianity has stated that the soul enters the scene at conception.

The Jehovah Witness thinks the body and the soul are the same thing.

Hindus believe in reincarnation so therefore, conception is when the soul begins its new life cycle.

Though opinions have varied at different points in history, those practicing Judaism maintain that the soul joins the body at birth and leaves at death.

There are those who believe the soul chooses its parents and family, [9] and hence, the idea the soul is present before conception. (So now if your kid gets mad at you for something, you can say, "Hey, *don't get upset. I read somewhere that kids pick their parents!")*

The reason for bringing up these ideas is to punch up the fact that most people on this planet believe that the soul is a separate entity from the physical body, and that the soul is the consciousness of the human person.

What's important here isn't whether the soul connects with the human body before, during or at birth. The main point is that the soul and the body are possibly not the same thing, and if that's the case, what exactly is the soul and what happens to it at body death?

Some believe they have a soul while others feel they are the soul.

I have talked with several women who have claimed that at more than one point during their pregnancy, they were awakened in the middle of the night or bombarded in their "space" at various times with spirits or souls who were noisily fighting each other over the possibility of taking possession of this new baby body.

Based on these claims, it appears that a disembodied soul considers a human body a highly desired commodity.

Another of my clients told me that when she was eight months pregnant, there was a moment late at night where she was awoken by a presence. It was a friendly but confident communication, "*I'm Gwendolyn*".

This spirit-soul was apparently informing my client that it not only intended on being the baby, but that the baby's name was to be Gwendolyn.

Because it was so unbelievable, she kept this event to herself.

The next day when she was at work, her boss came up to her and said, "*Hey, I was in a Walgreens late last night and I found these note-stickers that I bought for you.*

They say, "A Message from Gwendolyn". Isn't that the name you're giving your new baby?"

That very evening, she was attending a social event and a friend came up and said, "*I had a weird dream last night. Are you naming your baby Gwendolyn?*"

Looks like this Gwendolyn spirit was making the rounds, putting the word out and sealing the deal.

29.

When Does the Soul Leave the Body?

Like I mentioned earlier, it has been an observation that 21 grams of weight appears to leave a human body at death.

What is it that creates this weight and where does it go?

In some movies, there have been scenes where someone is dying, and the camera's viewpoint starts to move up and up and up, away from the dead body, as if it is an aware consciousness that is watching itself depart and separate from the shell it used to inhabit.

In the Star Wars story, Obi-Wan Kenobi tells Darth Vader, "*Vader, if you strike me down, I shall become more powerful than you can imagine.*" And once his dead body hits the ground, he's out, and is now everywhere.

One client told me that moments after her brother died she could perceive him on the ceiling of the hospital room, looking down on the scene. She was able to communicate with him telepathically and reassure him that everything would be okay.

Another client told me his wife had passed away at 1:30 P.M. in the oncology unit of a hospital. We'll call her Emily. Later that day, he said several people called and/

or texted him. One person was on the other side of the country, one was in an airplane and another one was in the same city but outside of the hospital. Each of these people asked something along the lines of, "*Did something happen to Emily around 1:30 today? I felt her with me at that moment.*" None of them were near Emily's bedside or anywhere near the hospital when she passed away. Yet all of them knew something happened and claimed they felt her with them at that exact time. It's as if at the moment of body death, she became *everywhere*.

30.

Break on Through to the Other Side

Tens of millions of people around the world have reported to having had a Near Death Experience (NDE).

This is when the body and/or brain have technically died, and the person later returns and tells what happened and what they experienced during the period of their so-called death.

There are many books and videos on this subject that detail remarkable similarities in all the stories that these people say they went through. A few of the descriptions include:

- Losing all pain
- Seeing a tunnel
- Following a light
- Dead relatives present to help transition back to life
- Love
- Calmness
- Reassurance
- Hope

Their overall perspective after such an experience seemed to generally take on some major shifts into what they now feel is important and what is not important in living their lives. I remember one talk where the speaker reported that many children who had an NDE, apparently became less concerned with school and normal educational subjects, but later took a huge interest in quantum physics which is a fundamental theory in physics which describes nature at the smallest scales of energy levels of atoms and subatomic particles. How about that?

Again, science doesn't have too much to say about all this because these phenomena and the stories told do not fit the current paradigm of the brain/consciousness model for explaining human life.

If the person you are helping starts talking or relating experiences similar to those descriptions I listed in this chapter, realize that millions of others on this planet share that same reality.

31.

Ghost in the Machine

If it is true that a ghost is the disembodied soul of a dead person, then what exactly are the specific parts that make up a living person?

Doesn't logic follow that if this so-called ghost phenomenon is happening and being experienced by over 145 million people over the history of this entire planet, maybe the Body-Mind-Spirit model is something that may be true or at least should be considered?

People have described and confided in me many incidents of so-called paranormal phenomena involving ghosts.

Here are a few shortened versions of what I have been told:

A 17-year-old girl was sleeping at her girlfriend's house. She was awoken in the middle of the night by a strange awareness that she was being watched. She opened her eyes and noticed her breath coming out of her mouth due to the huge drop of temperature that was now freezing cold by her bed. She started experiencing a heavy pressure on her chest as she was being pinned down to the bed.

This pushing continued and got heavier and heavier when an apparition of a man appears with his fingers bearing down on her. When she screamed and demanded he leave, everything went quiet. The pounding on her chest stopped and the temperature of that cold spot returned to normal.

The next morning, she told her girlfriend about this and the girlfriend admitted that she too had a similar experience in that same bedroom. She'd even invented a name for that man-ghost. George.

* * *

A woman I know once told me that when she was young, she was babysitting one night and fell asleep on the sofa. She soon felt a presence in front of her. When she opened her eyes, there was an old woman was sitting in a chair across the room staring at her.

Terrified, the girl closed her eyes but eventually opened them again. The chair was now empty.

The next day, she told her older sister about the phenomenon she'd encountered the night before and her sister said she too saw that same old ghost woman earlier when she was babysitting for that family, in that same house.

* * *

There was a house in the Midwest and I knew the family. Apparently, there were many reported instances of people hearing things being moved upstairs when no one else was home. When individuals would then go upstairs to investigate, all of the furniture was in a different position and the room was all messed up.

In that same house, one of the daughters was walking through the dining room, and all of a sudden, dishes and silverware from the shelves started flying across the room at her, smashing against the wall as she ducked and ran.

During holidays, kids would not play in one of the back areas of the house. When asked why they didn't play in that room, each said at separate times, *"There is a man back there and we don't like him."*

At a family reunion, a photo was taken in the house of all the people present. When the picture was developed, there was a little man in the photo who was not at that event and wasn't known by anyone in the family.

I saw that picture with my own eyes.

* * *

Another example was from a person who once told me that when he was younger, there had been this scary feeling near a spot under the stairs of their basement in the house where he and his family grew up. Every time someone would go down to the basement, a creepy, fearful emotion pervaded the space in this area. Eventually, it became apparent to those involved, that this emotion was coming from a ghost who had been the previous owner of the house but had died years ago. This spirit felt it was still his house and didn't want others to occupy it. A simple explanation and acknowledgement to this entity, regarding what had happened, ended the concern and that spirit left.

* * *

By including this section, I'm simply trying to punch up the fact that if the stories above are what people have told me, imagine how many other ghosts' experiences with other people there are out there around the planet. Try googling it and you'll see. It is just another one of those phenomena that is hard to explain but still is observed everywhere.

If a spirit without a body is what a ghost is, maybe the person at the end of life, whom you are now helping, is a spirit in a body, soon to be without a body.

Treat that concept with respect, even if not fully understood.

32.

Entities

"I hate when the voices in my head go silent.
I never know what they're planning."

The fact that someone wrote that phrase, and people always laugh at it when you say it, indicates there may be something to this whole arena.

Spirits, spirit-guides, deities, angels, Mara, Jezebel, entities, voices in the head, demons, spirit attachments, celestial beings, Gidim, fairies and mental circuits are some of the labels that have denoted a type of external "living" unit that appears to have influence over the lives of people.

Exorcism is the religious or spiritual practice of evicting demons or other types of entities from a person or location who is believed to be possessed. We've all seen the movie.

An associate of mine told me years ago he went to a psychic. He explained to this psychic that his estranged brother had died, and he was looking for some answers as to why his brother had acted the way he did and how his life had gotten so messed up.

During the session, this psychic explained that when his brother was alive, he had a "spiritual attachment" which had been an alcoholic during its life on earth and had forced his brother to drink and have an addictive personality.

A spiritual attachment?

There are people that claim they hear voices talking to them. Voices in their head.

In the story, "It's a Wonderful Life", Clarence, the angel, tells George Bailey that he has been a good influence towards the people he has been associated with.

Cupid is some entity that shoots a love arrow at a couple which gets them to fall in love so they'll procreate and carry on the race.

Fairies are believed to look out for our well-being.

Demons are evil and are feared as causing mental pain and confusion to those they target.

Black Magic, Voodoo, Witchcraft and Shamanism apparently attempt to evoke entities to carry out their spells and intentions. Supposedly, rituals and invocations are employed to bring forth these entities which are then utilized for the intended purposes of the conjurer.

Whether or not these things actually exist, or are just explanations for an observed type of phenomena, is something that can be debated. However, it is another topic that people talk about but science doesn't have a solid answer for. Therefore, you are within your rights to allow those you are helping to divulge their awarenesses and concerns if they start describing this type of thing to you. Just let them talk and don't shut them down.

33.

Placebo Effect

In the story "The Wizard of Oz", Dorothy wanted to get back to her Auntie Em (home), the Scarecrow wanted to be smart (a brain), the Tin Man wanted to have emotion (a heart) and the Lion wanted to stop being afraid (courage).

The Wizard told them he would help them, but first they had to prove themselves worthy by bringing him the broomstick of the Wicked Witch.

After a brilliant idea by the Scarecrow as to how to approach the witch's castle, the Tin Man's intuition as to where Dorothy was located, and because of the fighting ability and heightened aggressiveness of the Lion, they were successful in their mission and returned to the Wizard with the broomstick.

This is where the Wizard pointed out to each of them that they were already endowed with the abilities they were hoping to achieve, but that up until now, they had not yet stepped up and displayed or acknowledged what they inherently possessed.

Even Dorothy realized that if she was ever to seek true happiness, she didn't have to look any further than her own backyard. In other words, *herself*.

Throughout history, including the New Age movements in the 1970's and 1980's, there have been those individuals who would always purport that you have untapped potential:

- *"There is no man living who isn't capable of doing more than he thinks he can do."* (Henry Ford)
- *"Awaken the giant within."* (Tony Robbins)
- *"Our deepest fear is not that we are inadequate. Our deepest fear is that we are powerful beyond measure."* (Marianne Williamson)

Necessity will often bring out an increase in human ability. There are so many examples of individuals rising above adversity and physical limitations when there is an urgency or higher purpose present. People have been known to perform unreal and impossible feats of strength when no other option presented itself. Like the mothers who have lifted a car up with one arm and pulled their son or daughter out from under it with the other arm.

In her book *"One Hundred Hearts"* author Terry Sidford lists scores of stories and examples of people being able to rise up out of horrible, seemingly impossible life circumstances due to nothing more than an absolute necessity, which then brought about renewed abilities and perseverance that had previously been absent.

Come on, "mind over matter" is a well-known phrase.

Millions claim that praying to a God, that can't be physically seen, benefits them in their life.

Doctors have told me that some patients don't get better

no matter what procedures or medications are prescribed. Science acknowledges the fact that some people improve their medical condition simply by taking sugar pills. Science doesn't know why it works.

Hope alone can bring some people out of an emotional depression.

There is a word, "*Entelechy*":

(*Aristotelian metaphysics*) The complete realization and final form of some potential concept or function: the conditions under which a potential thing becomes actualized.

(*Chiefly philosophy*) A particular type of motivation, need for self-determination, and inner strength directing life and growth to become all one is capable of being: the need to actualize one's beliefs: having both a personal vision and the ability to actualize that vision from within.

Do we all have the same dynamic drive to succeed? The same fears? Aggressions? Complacency? Abilities? Problem-solving skills?

The answer is obviously no.

Determining what exactly is the catalyst for change in another person is just not a quantifiable proposition. How much was it the pill that caused the improvement? Was it the attention given, the suggested advice or the instructions that created the change? What percentage of the remedy involved the "will" of the patient or client?

When dealing with someone who is dying, their mental state and outlook are often a greater influence on their well being than any further surgeries or medical handling. Confidence that their wishes will be carried out, purging themselves of guilt and regret, hope that they will continue in some capacity after body death and the reassurance that everyone around them will be okay, all play a role in their physical condition. The amount of pain and upset they will either have or not have, as they live out their remaining time here, probably depends on their ideological perspective more than anything else.

I have even seen a method to alleviate sickness that at the outset seems totally ridiculous. If you want to help someone with an illness or condition that keeps persisting, just give them a bunch of attention. Have them on an impossible regimen that you prescribe. Help them to move their bed to the north wall so the sun will be maximumly present for 3 hours in their room. Tell them to drink half a cup of water, every 2 hours but nothing between 4:00 pm and 7:00 pm. Tell them to take 3 blue pills (all sugar pills) on every odd numbered day and 2 yellow pills twice a day on every even numbered day... but skip Thursdays.

Just the fact that they are getting that much attention sometimes can remove their feelings of isolation or desperation and now their physical symptoms seem to lesson as a result. Or, being sick was just a means of getting attention and since that purpose has now been achieved, they no longer must "hold on" to their illness.

In the movie, "The Invention of Lying", the main character's mother is dying. She is in a hospital bed, with total fear, crying, saying she is terrified that she will be thrown into a darkness of nothing for eternity. Her son is so upset at seeing his mom this way that he immediately thinks up a story and he tells her that no, she has it wrong. He explains to her that she actually will be going to a beautiful place, where there is love and harmony, and there'll be a mansion waiting for her and she can dance again like when she was young. She smiles, contemplating the possibility of this reality and dies right then and there. Peacefully.

What is wrong with a sugar pill if the effects are the same as the medically approved cure? What is wrong with blowing off medical procedures and surgery if comfort, dignity and acceptance of mortality are a bigger priority than scientific facts?

Doctors are put in a stressful position when people at the end of life are asking what they should do. Should I have the operation? Should I go through chemo treatments again? What will my chances of recovery be? How much longer will I live if I go through the operation? What will be the side effects? What happens if I don't have the surgery?

How can a medical doctor know the answers to all these questions? He can't. There are too many factors out of his control. Asking him how much time grandma has left to live is also difficult because some of that answer has to do with grandma herself.

I have seen people with injuries and illnesses return to health almost immediately when they were asked a certain type of question. The Progressive Question, mentioned in a later chapter. This type of question can help uncover unconscious decisions or past conclusions that can actually hold an illness or injury in place and prevent recovery.

* * *

One client of mine had a really bad cold, watery eyes, red face and a runny nose for days.

After one question, asked and answered, suddenly, his eyes cleared up, his nose stopped running and his redness went away.

One question.

* * *

Another client accidentally cut his thumb off in a band saw accident. He was in the hospital, cast applied, a pin was placed through the thumb, and he was being monitored daily. The doctors were unsure if he would ever regain functional use of his thumb again.

I visited him in the hospital and after I asked one of these progressive type questions, he hit something in his mind. His skin got flushed, his eyes opened wide, and he relayed this huge epiphany relating to how this injury occurred and how he now saw how the injury was serving him in some crazy, unconscious way.

The next day the doctors couldn't believe it. His thumb had completely fused back together, and life had been fully restored in it. My client was a guitarist and a couple weeks later, he went back out on tour.

* * *

A woman I was counseling had been trying to get pregnant for years. She and her husband had been through all the physical tests and hormone treatments but nothing was happening. After a series of these types of progressive questions, she all of a sudden spotted a negative decision about having children that she had made as a very, very young girl. She'd formed this decision during a moment of heavy trauma when she witnessed her parents fighting violently.

That next month she missed her period, and now they have three children.

* * *

I've spoken with healthcare professionals that have all said there are some patients that just don't recover as most other patients do with the same symptoms and treatments. Why is that? Could it be that something mentally or spiritually is holding back their recovery?

Do not discount the fact that attitude, belief, outlook, necessity, and other factors are at play when you are providing aid to someone. The unexplained Placebo Effect can at least be acknowledged and as something that exists for some, including those at the end of life.

Section Five

HARD CORE SOFT SKILLS

It is evident that with the advancement of technology and social media, the ability to have a meaningful, face-to-face conversation with another person has almost become a lost art.

34.

Anything Powerful is Simple

If your uncle tells you he wants to die, what will you say? How will you deal with it? How will you coach others around your uncle to react to those types of realities?

When you are helping someone in any capacity, you'll need to have some command over communication, sensitivity, and an awareness of how to engage with another person.

This section is included simply because when you are helping someone who is dying, you'll want to know what to expect and how to act accordingly. This skill will also help to keep things as smooth as possible, including reactions and requests from all the family and friends who will be present.

I call these "Hard Core Soft Skills".

Hard: Because these core skills are so basic and such an integral part of everything they are often hard to notice, explain and utilize.

Core: Most of them are very fundamental and are the core of what's underneath all successful interpersonal relationships.

Soft Skills: Personal attributes that enable someone to

interact effectively and harmoniously with other people.

Anything powerful is usually very simple. Hopefully, these chapters will shed some light on effective ways to approach communication when helping someone pass away peacefully, and in your own life for that matter.

35.

Help!

If you take a look and do a breakdown on the subject of helping others, you'll see a few common aspects:

- You have two or more people involved.
- You'll need to utilize some form of communication
- You should establish whether that person actually wants help
- What is it that the other considers to be true help?

There are other factors too.

Assuming you already know what a person needs before actually establishing what they really want, often results in trouble.

I remember someone telling me that a woman she knew was a devout Christian Scientist. This religion holds a belief which views the physical world as an illusion and maintains that the only reality is the spiritual world. It also purports that Jesus Christ came to provide spiritual and physical healing by correcting our wrong perceptions in this illusion; Sickness and illnesses being one of these "errors in perception". Therefore, going to a doctor in search of a physical cure would be diametrically opposed to that belief system and would only fuel the fire of this "error."

When she eventually became old and very ill, some of her children and grandchildren pleaded with her to seek medical attention. She refused and requested that they respect her by keeping the doctors away, because it violated what she believed and wanted.

She did not consider that going to the doctor was a form of help.

Well, they didn't listen to her wishes. An ambulance was called; she got strapped into a gurney and was shuffled off to a hospital, where she spent her remaining days in misery and hopelessness because of being forced into a situation that she opposed.

The so-called help that was dumped on her was a betrayal of what she considered true help. Help of a religious and spiritual nature.

Parents do this all the time. Their child is trying to tie his shoe and the parent says, *"Let me help you with that"*, and proceeds to grab the kid's shoelaces. The child gets really upset and screams out, *"I wanted to do it!"*

You don't want your help to create another problem.

People in pain and/or dying sometimes just want to be left alone. Help would mean allowing them to remain undisturbed for a period of time. Having others present in the room and having to listen to what they have to say is often too stressful. Maybe just sitting with them silently would be what they need and want. If you set yourself up as a person they can be totally honest with, they will tell you what help they actually want.

When you're attempting to provide aid to someone, make sure you are in tune with what they consider true help is for them. You do this by asking questions, listening and not asserting what you think real help should be or what you think they need.

36.

Presence

Have you ever been talking to someone and they are staring at their phone or watching something else, not looking at you? Have you ever told someone something and they reacted so badly that you wished you'd never said anything? How about when you were a teenager, and your parents asked you where you were, who you were there with and what you'd been up to, and when you gave your answers, they immediately started scolding and reprimanding you for what you just told them? I bet the next time they asked where you were, you probably said something like "*the library*".

Interpersonal relationships do well when things can flow without recourse, harshness, counter-attacks or inattention.

Being fully present helps accomplish this.

Some examples of situations that drag us out of being present in the moment:

- Someone is bleeding and you freak out over seeing the blood. You then won't be a very trusted source of help to that person. They'd rather have someone who can assess the situation and act correctly without emotion and fear.

- You are in a bar and need to help a buddy who has had too much to drink. In the past you got sick drinking tequila and you smell it now, react, feel sick to your stomach, and are not be able to be fully present in the actual moment to help your friend. You are somewhat stuck in that earlier time and what is happening right now isn't being fully experienced.

- Someone dumped you in the past and the person you are talking to now, tells you they just got dumped. This may trigger your past loss and that unpleasant memory, which then means you are not fully listening to what that person is saying to you now.

- You are trying to complete a project, but you are constantly thinking about some life problem or what you must do tomorrow. Your attention is not on your current action and it is doubtful that you will get much done on that project today.

When you react badly to what someone says or does, some interesting things happen. Your disapproval or upset will shut down further communications from them.

When someone is yelling, we tend to only recognize the fact that they are mad, and thus the words they are sputtering out don't have much meaning other than they are pissed. If you show aggressive or disturbing emotions, anything you claim or any point you are trying to make will get discounted as "you're just upset".

It is normally easier to deal with a problem when there are two people working shoulder to shoulder to resolve it. Figuring out solutions on your own is sometimes difficult. This is why we tell people about situations in our life. Two-way communication is a powerful tool to help get our heads out of the confusing situation and look at it from different angles and viewpoints.

When you react badly to what someone is saying, you become part of the problem and now that person must deal with the problem, plus your reactions, thus no more shoulder to shoulder. Your reaction and the problem are now shoulder to shoulder against that person.

When you ask a question, you are the one initiating the communication. You are the one in control. If you are coaching someone, raising kids or in charge of a project, you'll want to maintain some control and direction, so you can steer it to the correct result. When you react to what someone says or does, they are in fact controlling the communication because they initiated something that you reacted to, so they are now "running the show" by default. If you lose the lead, you'll lose the ability to bring about the intended and desired result.

* * *

So, what is presence? It's being able to be in a space comfortably and taking in all that is happening without anything else going on with you, mentally or physically. Undisturbed observation. The mind tends to compulsively throw things at us during our life, which then obscures the true scene in front of us and prevents an appropriate or effective response.

Maintaining presence, or being 100% present during communication and/or events that occur, allows problems to get resolved much easier than including your reactions in the mix. Try it next time. Next time you feel yourself getting worked up by what someone says or does, try just being completely present with their communication and that's all. You'd be amazed at how much quicker things can get settled when you can maintain a composed presence.

When you're helping someone with these steps, do whatever you need to do to practice having a calm and inviting presence. Tensions and emotions tend to be at a high point with everyone involved, so maintain a safe and reassuring demeanor, without biased reactions.

Everyone will really appreciate the fact that "someone's got it together" during this trying time.

37.

Accept "What Is"

Protesting something you wish was not true doesn't do anything but make it worse.

The first step in dealing with anything in life is looking at the real scene in front of you. Then you can plan out how to help it, improve it, or leave it alone.

There are realities you may have to face, when helping individuals at the end of life, which may not be pleasant. Pain, unconsciousness, grief, medical devices, drugs, tubes, bad smells, incoherent communications and general overwhelm are some of the things you'll have to deal with.

The only way to effectively deal with it is to accept it without back off.

Jim Collins wrote a book called, "Good to Great". It was a study of companies that went from an average level and rose to a quality level of greatness. Collin's team studied everything in these companies from their leadership, to how they hired and placed people in positions at the company. They also investigated the overall philosophy the company stood for, how they conducted their meetings, the decision-making process and what pieces of technology they should implement to forward their purposes.

One of the biggest discoveries is outlined in a chapter called, *"Confront the Brutal Facts"*. The leaders of these great companies never became fixed and stuck on anything regarding what they were doing or the processes they utilized. They were flexible enough to improve their business model to fit what was really happening around them all the time.

They would continually look into what the public wanted, where the market was heading, how their customers were responding and how they could continue to improve and expand in their ever-changing environment.

When you are helping others, confronting the brutal facts is also a good idea to strive for. Do not try to push away unpleasant realities. Don't pretend it is different than it is. Trying to force something into a more comfortable actuality, will not work in the long run.

This is an important Hard Core Soft Skill because this one is the foundation underlying everything else you'll do.

Be present, accept what is, listen and then help, is the sequence that will give you the greatest chance of success in aiding the dying person and his or her families.

38.

Listen

"Listening is such a simple act. It requires us to be present, and that takes practice, but we don't have to do anything else. We don't have to advise, or coach, or sound wise. We just have to be willing to sit there and listen."

(Wheatley)

Easier said than done. Especially when confronted with the subject of death.

If your grandfather is lying there and tells you "... *It's time*", can you listen without falling apart?

As a coach, as a counselor, or in life, staying in the "now" and listening is extremely important if you want to be effective in helping another person.

Being the receipt of bad, ugly or hard-to face communication or situations should be received without anything other than acknowledging the fact that you have received it.

I've seen this with parents raising kids. The parent asks their child a question. The kid answers, and the parent reacts and rants on and on about the answer they just heard. As mentioned earlier, the next time you ask your kid for the truth, good luck.

If you are assisting someone with a serious condition, and it brings to mind a bad threat, loss or experience, and you start obsessing over that earlier time, it will be hard for you to listen, be effective and provide aid to the person in front of you now.

Communication heals. If no one is listening, only limited healing is taking place.

Many have written about the idea of "being in the Now". The idea that there is no past or future, only Now, is a good model to follow to help you be present without fear, trepidation, worry or back off. Anyone who wants to be more effective in their life needs to be fully present in any situation, without being dragged out of it by the mind's compulsive thinking process. When you are helping someone else, being present and fully listening is the best and fastest way to obtain results.

Another difficulty in all this is the fact that listening means being the *receipt* of a communication. Sometimes being the receipt of things is something we don't like and even despise. Like getting hit in the face, having a past due bill arrive in the mail, receiving a bad report card, having a policeman handing you a speeding ticket, developing an illness, getting fired, being dumped by a girlfriend, boy-friend or spouse, problems, upsets and every other unde-sirable aspect of life of which we are on the receiving end.

Receiving starts to leave a bad taste in our mouths.

Have you ever run into people who can't receive anything you say to them? You tell them you went to Yellowstone National Park for a vacation, and they go off on how their trip to Maui was so much more incredible and blabber on and on to the point you wished you'd never even brought up the subject?

Or, you mention an accomplishment and they start defending themselves on why they haven't been able to pull off a similar feat:

You: *"I ran a 10K last weekend."*

Them: *"Oh yeah, well... I strained a hamstring a while back and my doctor wants me to take it easy for the rest of the year, otherwise I would have been running in that thing too. In fact, a couple years ago I was running a half marathon and I blah, blah, blah..."*

They just don't want to be on the receiving end of anything. They become compulsive on talking so that you can't put them in a position of having to listen, because listening means receiving and receiving means, "Bad! Stay away".

When you listen to someone, you're giving him or her a chance to describe what is going on with them, allowing them to tell you what their attention is on and what they would consider as help. Giving advice is okay but telling someone what they should do without having fully listened and clarified what is really going on, will be less effective in bringing about an improved condition all the way around.

It is very important to effectively listen when providing aid to someone. Practice meditation techniques, counseling, walking, exercise, quiet time in nature or whatever means you can utilize to slow down your thinking process so you can be present and listen.

Start being aware and make a conscious effort to listen in your normal, everyday conversations. Make sure the person has said all they want to say before you interject. Ask people questions and really listen. Practice showing care and empathy by being interested in what others are doing or feeling or communicating. Let people know that what they said meant something to you with an appropriate acknowledgement to what they just told you. Don't judge, listen. Observe the person in front of you to the point that you know how to make them feel comfortable and safe enough to tell you anything.

Any difficulty with relationships can probably be traced to someone, somewhere not listening.

Remember, someone whose body is ill or dying may not be able to respond as quickly as you're accustom to. You need to wait and make sure that they have communicated everything they want to say. Sometimes they can't even speak verbally or might be slurring their words, so your "listening" may consist only of observation and picking up on what they wish they could say.

39.

Don't Overdo Any Step

I'm sure you can recall times when someone was explaining something to you and then suddenly, boom, you understood completely what they were talking about... but they just kept going on and on and on. Or, a salesman is enthusiastically detailing how awesome his product is and somewhere during his sales pitch you actually have the thought that you should buy it, and you're happy with that decision, but he doesn't pick up on this and keeps blabbering to the point you tell him that you'll have to think about it and then you leave without purchasing anything. How about when you're sick and someone provides you with some relief or comfort but then continues trying to help to the point of annoyance?

In other words, they just don't know when to stop.

I call this going past the "point of payoff" (POP). This hard core soft skill is something to be aware of in all of your interpersonal relationships but especially important when you're dealing with someone who is very ill or at the end of life.

These directives may be taxing on someone who is dying. Be sensitive to this fact by only doing as many steps at one sitting as required, without the person becoming exhausted or overwhelmed.

Thinking and communicating is sometimes hard. You should have a short-term goal for each step of the program.

If you're doing the step where you are asking for a list of people to which grandma wants a message relayed, and she seems satisfied with the list, end off for that period of time. If you push any step past a desirable point, tiredness usually sinks in and they may become agitated or upset.

Set the goal of the person being better off than when you entered the room and once you've achieved that, end off for that that period of time.

Be aware of any subtle changes, a sigh, breathing better, a slight smile, or a sign of contentment. Maintain communication as you go along and coax them to always let you know how they are feeling during this period of time you are helping them.

To ensure you don't overdo anything, give a few moments for the person to respond to your directives and questions. This will give them a chance to answer and also allows you to make sure you're tracking with them so you'll know when to end off at a good point.

40.

It's the Question

How are you going to help someone if you don't know what he or she needs?

Ask questions. That's how.

There is an entire philosophy in sales where you should be asking questions 90% of the time to be successful.

It seems there has been a recent effort of companies, managers and professionals to start incorporating better questions into the mix of their operations.

Even Albert Einstein once said: *"If I had an hour to solve a problem and my life depended on the solution, I would spend the first 55 minutes determining the proper question to ask, for once I know the proper question, I could solve the problem in less than five minutes"*.

I once heard that our main drive in life is to create; create anything that can be seen, experienced and acknowledged, good or bad. Apparently, the fundamental reason to be alive is to produce something that we can present to others and ourselves.

The child brings you a picture he painted. A musician writes a piece of music he loves and hopes others will. The young girl describes her awesome European vacation. The older man buys a sports car so others will see him in it. A wife displays frustration so her husband will know the importance of what she is aware of.

We like it best when we create something and the other person receives it as we'd intended. We don't like it when we can't get our point across or our creation isn't understood or worse, simply ignored.

It's like that old scenario:

Her: *"I just don't think you really care about me anymore."*

Him: *"I'm sorry... were you saying something?"*

In this light, asking a question is powerful, because you are allowing another to show you or present to you what they want you to see or be aware of. The question prompts another to show you what they want you to know. In other words, it aligns with this basic purpose in us all.

If the child cries and you ignore her, she'll cry harder. You're just not getting the severity of what she's trying to show you. If you ask a question like, *"What's wrong?"*, your child can explain, and if you now say, *"Oh, I get it."*, she will have at least accomplished the short-term goal of ensuring you know what she is upset about.

You won't know unless you ask.

You: *"Hi grandma. How are you feeling today, as compared to yesterday?"*

Grandma: *"Well, I had a bit of nausea this morning, but I slept better last night and feel less pressure in my arms now. Seems like everything is a bit better."*

You: *"That's good to hear".*

You see? Because of your question, she was able to achieve the purpose of you now understanding what she wanted you to know.

This is so basic that it is often hard to isolate and it just goes by unnoticed. But it's the key to successful interpersonal relationships and life.

A woman stands in front of a mirror for 5 minutes, looking at the blouse she is going to wear, hoping it looks good to others, and then at the party, someone walks up and says, *"Hey, I like your blouse. Looks great. Where did you get it?"* Boom! She smiles because she pulled off what she was hoping to create.

Simple.

Allow others to let you know what they want you to know by asking them questions. By doing this, you'll be able to help in a big way.

Giving advice doesn't do this. When you give someone advice, you're putting them in a position to have to listen to what you are trying to create, and it doesn't fulfill their underlying intentions.

As far as giving advice goes, here's something else to be aware of. Offering advice is fine if someone has a question as to how to do something that you are knowledgeable in.

- *"What's a good chili recipe?"*
- *"How do you enroll for this class online?"*

- *"Do you know of a competent electrician?"*
- *"Is there a dating website that you heard was good?"*
- *"Who won the 2016 Super Bowl?"*

If you know the answers to those types of questions, go for it. Give your advice or recommendations. People can also look for those types of answers on Google, YouTube and Wikipedia.

But when someone has a personal problem like:

- *"My husband is mean and abusive to me."*
- *"My job sucks."*
- *"I feel depressed all the time."*
- *"My teenager is out of control."*
- *"What will happen when I die?"*

You'll be better off staying away from giving advice and switch to the power of the question.

What is behind the problem they are telling you? How was it constructed and what is the architecture under it? What are all the possible ins and outs and details that could exist about that problem?

You probably have no idea or could only assume to know. A dicey proposition.

Let's list out a few possibilities of what could be underneath and around the problem, *"My husband is mean and abusive to me"*:

- Emotional pain.
- Physical pain.

- Confusions and overwhelm.

- Memories of similar problems.

- The players in this particular problem (her parents, his parents, kids, friends etc.).

- The relationships between all the players.

- The agreements between all these players.

- How long the problem has existed.

- Secrets and lies within and around this situation.

- Her part in creating this problem.

- His part in it.

- How might this problem be serving her.

It should be obvious why blurting out some advice on this one has virtually no chance of resolving it. Your recommendation would never "hit the nail on the head" because there are about 100 nails around, throughout and within this problem.

She tells you her husband is abusive, and you blurt out, *"Well, you should leave him. Divorce him!"*

I figure there are basically four possible reactions to your advice on a situation like this (and by the way, the first one listed below will *never* happen):

1. She says, *"Oh my God! You're a genius! I can't believe I never thought of that. Yeah, I should leave him! Thank you so much. I'm gonna do it!"* And she does.

2. She apathetically says something like, *"Yeah, you're probably right. I guess I should leave him. Yeah... Well,*

I'll talk to you later." Another two weeks goes by and nothing has changed.

3. She gets pissed at you. She angrily asserts, *"Oh yeah, right. And what about the kids? They love him. Am I supposed to just rip their dad away from them? And where am I supposed to go? I mean, he makes money and I don't make that much. What do you want me to do... Go live with my mother? I'd rather drink battery acid than to go back and live with my mother! I can't believe you are so over-simplistic. You can't possibly understand what I'm going through!"*

4. (And this is the worst one) She comes back to you a couple weeks later and sheepishly says, *"Well I took your advice. My husband and I got into a big argument the other night, and I told him what you said. I let him know that you think I should divorce him. But ya know, he's actually a good guy, and I really do love him, and he says he'll stop going to those strip clubs, and he promised to cut down on his drinking, and... oh yeah, he said he wants to talk to you."*

There is a certain type of question that I have used for years in my coaching and counseling. It is designed to get a person look at things in a new way, without me having to give advice or tell them anything.

I call it a "Progressive Question" because it can help someone progress from one level of awareness, and increase it to a higher, more expanded and logical degree of awareness. This type of question or directive can shed light on old decisions that are holding someone back, false fears, limiting considerations and potential-killing withdrawal from reaching for one's goals. In other words, an increased awareness of life.

Increased awareness gives an increase of choice.

In the example above, you could ask questions like:

"How long has this been going on?"

"What type of abuse have you been experiencing?

When and how often does this normally occur?"

"Who else knows about this?"

"How have you reacted to it?"

"When did it start?"

"Did something happen prior that may have contributed to this behavior?"

"What solutions have you been considering regarding it"

"Have you ever seen this type of situation before, in yours' or someone else's life?

Questions like these can help the other person to look at the scene they are in and see it from various angles, which then provides a much greater chance of them unraveling and resolving their particular situation far better than any advice you could dream up.

Even a simple step like having someone take a walk and look at things in their surroundings until they feel better can help pop them out of doubts, fears and confusion into a more calm and stable state-of-mind.

Asking someone to remember something in his or her life, is actually automatically pointing out the fact that there is a difference between back when it happened and now. A powerful process.

If the person at the end of life is acting afraid, sometimes asking something like, *"Can you remember ever being scared like this in the past?"* can actually help them to spot the fact that those past fears may be contributing to their current state, and therefore, just using that simple question can de-intensify the unpleasant emotion he or she is currently feeling.

You could say that most of the steps in this book have the purpose of helping the dying person feel better, less fearful and more "grounded" by the end of that particular step than they did at the beginning of it.

Asking someone to look around the room until they appear brighter, or have them talk about their accomplishments in life, or list out all the people they want to get a message delivered to, can be considered a valid progressive question or directive.

Anything you do or ask which brings about a fresher outlook, creates a sense of closure, produces less anxiety and/or a feeling that they have accomplished something, is a legitimate coaching step. Any activity that gets them to progress from an anxious worry to a calm satisfaction is a correct action and should be done.

Questions can help in a big way. Use them.

41.

Be Effective

Okay, so sympathy has its place, but when you are in a serious situation, you'd rather have someone competent helping you through it.

There will be plenty of people around the dying person who will be exuding sympathy. There won't be a shortage of that, although you should try to prevent them from pouring it on too much. The person at the end-of life might not like everyone continually reminding them of their own mortality.

Come on, if you were sitting there bleeding, would you want a paramedic, with all their knowledge and equipment, to administer the correct action, apply the right bandage and give the right medications, or would you prefer to have them stand there and tell you how sorry they are that you are in such a bad situation? *"I'm so sorry. I feel so bad for you..."*

If you take on the role of helping someone at the end of life, keep the attitude pleasant but effective. You are dealing with a real person, like you, so lay off the syrupy, sympathetic emotions and take control of the situation. Remove confusion; provide stability, guidance and hope.

Instead of being affected, be effective.

42.

Help the Person in Front of You

The help provided to someone at the end of life, or in any circumstance, must be administered with common sense and reality.

If grandpa is blind, don't ask him to look out the window at the trees.

The point is, use judgment and decide what and how you are going to use this information based on the scene in front of you. Pick out the steps you feel confident in applying.

I have noticed in my days as a coach and counselor, that some respond differently than others.

Gather information about the environment, condition of the person, what the hospice or medical personnel advise and what the family and friends have witnessed thus far.

Like I said, doing anything on that list of steps is better than doing nothing, but the more you can tailor these steps to the person you're in front of, the better.

Remember, don't expect them to answer a question or carry out a directive, unless you know they are able to do so.

There are few other things to keep in mind when you're engaged in helping a person at the end of life.

It is interesting to note that the last few days of life may possibly be the point where a person will experience more clarity then they have ever had in their entire lifetime. The "urge to survive" can cause people to be and do many things that may not align with who they really are, or what they actually believe, or truly desire. Like, having to work a dead-end job just for the money. Staying in a toxic relationship because it seems there are no other options, or not doing the things you love because you've set your life up to be consumed with everything that has the appearance of keeping you and others alive, but little to do with who you really are.

When surviving is no longer a driving force, a person can experience and remember what has been buried up by a lifetime of compromise.

In light of this, you'll need to acknowledge and grant the dying person the status of having a quality overview and grasp of knowing what's important in life and what's actually not that important in the overall scheme of things.

Just because they cannot respond and/or communicate as quickly as normal, doesn't mean they are not aware. Their physical limitations don't necessarily indicate that their cognitive abilities have also stopped.

Being present, asking questions and listening are the best ways to establish knowing the person in front of you and what they consider important, which in turn, enables your help to be effective and appreciated.

43.

Hard Core Soft Skills Summary

(As applicable to helping someone at the end of life)

1. Help the person in front of you.

2. Ask questions.

3. Listen.

4. Be present without reactions.

5. Don't force your beliefs or ideas.

6. Avoid giving advice.

7. Allow them to be who they are without judgment.

8. Don't assume you know. Communicate.

9. Don't make agreements you can't keep.

10. Assess the scene you're confronted with and act accordingly.

11. Don't overdo any step. Use a light approach. Always try to end at a good point.

12. Don't ask something that cannot be answered or carried out.

13. Refrain from exuding too much sympathy. Be compassionate but effective.

14. Work as a team with any family member, hospice personnel or medical staff.

Section Six

EVERY LITTLE THING

Further Guidelines and Recommendations

44.

To Nursing and Hospice Professionals

The advice in this book is in no way intended to conflict with those in the medical or hospice professions. My wish is that some of these steps may complement the care and tools that are already being utilized.

A paramedic has had to confront things that I can only imagine. A doctor in the ER trying to keep someone alive by applying pressure to a bleeding artery is something I have never dealt with. A hospice nurse holding the hand of a previous stranger as they die, but who has spent the last several weeks at their bedside, caring for, keeping them comfortable, providing food and medications, engaging in intimate, reassuring discussions, and having grown to love them, is an emotional reality most of us have not had to face.

I have been able to help ease some of the fear and confusion for those that are dying and thus, augment the professional services being provided by others. Any of these recommendations can be employed or handpicked as seen fit.

Healthcare staff can also provide the information contained herein to the friends and family on the scene so they can help make their loved one more comfortable. They will listen to a professional. Giving them something effective to do, rather than sitting around the bed staring at their grandpa, will benefit them greatly.

People love to help and provide value. Agitation, upsets and problems often come about when a person feels he or she can't do anything about a situation. Allowing those around the dying person a chance to do something meaningful for their loved one will help everyone involved. Nursing and hospice staff included.

45.

To Religious and Spiritual Advisers

There are no attempts here to force any faith, belief system or religion. A coach is there to help, not judge.

If the person at the end of life has been attending a particular church or temple, a representative from that religion is in the best position to offer strength and reassurance throughout his or her last days.

It's my hope that some of this information can work hand and hand with religious advisors and their counseling.

As I stated earlier, this advice can be delegated to others to perform as applicable. Simple directions given to the friends and family will give purpose and the satisfaction that comes from helping. *"Please go in and ask your grandpa if there is anything at his house that he would like brought here to his room in the hospital and make a list so we can help him out."* or any version of this kind of thing will do wonders for the morale of the family members.

Because these requests are coming from someone they trust and have faith in, it will mean that much more.

46.

You May Need to Coach the Coach

There may be instances where you will need to instruct someone else to carry out this information and these steps. Maybe the dying would feel more comfortable and trusting of someone else, especially a person they are familiar with. If so, let them. You can be behind the scene helping the helper.

Many times there will be one main family member who has taken on the role as the representative to the doctors or hospice personnel. I have often observed that it's the oldest daughter that is the one catering to the needs of her dying parent. She will be the one to whom everybody close to the dying person is listening to and looking for guidance as to what is happening throughout the process. At any rate, make sure your actions are coordinated to contribute and be accepted as help to the individual who has taken on that responsibility. This could very well be the person most able to coach their loved one with these steps.

Instead of you dealing directly with the person at the end of life, you can help as a consultant to the one who has been taking charge and who everyone trusts. Best to have them read through this book and then you both can plan out the steps they'll be taking. Sometimes it helps to have another person in the background supervising the coach because he or she can remain objective and act as a guide.

Most of the stories and examples you are reading here are instances of me coaching someone who was actually applying these steps, face to face, with someone they were close to. In fact, there have been many times when I heard someone mentioning that their loved one was in a hospital, dying, and all I said was, *"There are a couple things I'm aware of that you can do to help them."* Just that statement alone meant the world to them. The fact that there was somebody who knew something they could do to help, was a huge relief all by itself. They no longer felt alone in their situation. I would then describe or email them some of the directives in this book and tell them to call me at any point and let me know how things were going. They were so thankful to have someone who understood what they were dealing with and could talk with openly.

Don't underestimate the help you can provide.

You can be a coach to the coach and be a reassuring presence throughout the process.

47.

If You Know You Know

There is an aspect to all this I want to drive home.

When eminent death is present, emotions are elevated and people tend to get very overwhelmed and upset. Even the calmest personalities may break down when faced with a loved one on his or her deathbed. The family and friends around this dying person generally will not know what to do or say in this situation. There will be arguments, crying, guilt, confusion, financial stress, disagreements on what is to be done and general apathy.

In a traumatic event, whoever takes charge will be followed by the rest.

When someone is dying, no one in and around the family generally has a handle as to what's going on, and they will be relieved when somebody else steps up and starts giving direction. Consult who you need to and don't over-step your welcome, but if you know what to do, do it.

Hospice staff, doctors, nurses, medical personnel and social workers are there to do what they do best, but the family members around the injured, ill or dying, often make it very difficult. In addition to the jobs these professionals are there to perform, there is often a constant questioning of their every move, unreasonable requests, and non-stop badgering.

There will also be those who will just remain as spectators and assume everyone else is going to help grandma through it. Realize that there are certain aspects of providing aid to someone on their deathbed that you now are becoming aware of. So, once you know what you can do to help, go ahead and start helping. Just like raising your children, there is really no one else that can do that. If you acknowledge this fact, you can be effective. Don't assume someone else is going to know what to do to help the dying person pass away peacefully.

Realize that in a stressful situation, if you can respond in a positive manner, others will be thankful that you do.

Another thing. Don't wait until the last breath of life. Try to establish yourself as someone who can help as early as possible. If you are aware of someone going through medical procedures that may or may not resolve a prolonged life, go and see them and provide some assistance as best you can. If you can connect on some level at this point, when it comes to those last days, you'll be a trusted source of comfort.

If someone you know has a loved one who is at the point where he or she may be close to body death, help coach them with what you know so they can provide assistance, before it's too late.

People tend to wait until there are so many operations and drugs involved that communication and reassurance becomes difficult.

Recently an acquaintance of mine heard that I was working on this book and she contacted me. Her husband's grandpa was dying, and they were on the way to the hospital to see him. She asked for advice as to what they could do.

Not knowing anything of his condition or the environment he was in, I gave some simple instructions along the lines of:

1. Try to spend a few moments alone with your grandfather.

2. Hold his hand as a reference point for him.

3. Thank him for anything he contributed to your life.

4. Find out if there is anything he needs taken care of, or any messages he wants delivered to anyone.

5. Find out what he feels the next "chapter" holds for him.

Well, it turns out that this grandpa had been battling cancer for the last three years, including numerous medical procedures, chemo drips and radiation treatments. He was now on morphine and pretty much out of it. My acquaintance said she could only do those first three steps because her grandfather was going in and out of consciousness, but she was so very grateful for the direction she was given. She said prior to this, she had no idea what to do under these types of circumstances. She was also relieved that she was given a good approach to say goodbye to her grandpa.

Make contact as early as possible and do whatever steps make sense as time goes on. If you wait until the last day or so, you may be limited in the help you can give.

Even if you did just one of the things listed in this book, it would go a long way toward helping your loved one. With a good heart, you really can't mess anything up. Please just be the coach. Get going! Walk into the room, and tell everyone else to give you a few minutes alone with (dying person's name). Straighten things up. Have him or her touch a few things to get oriented. Ask what they're worried about. Let them know you're "on it". Tell them they did great with their life and everyone is appreciative of all they've given.

Let them know that at any point they decide it's time to let go of their body, it is totally their decision to do so and that you'll make sure everyone else is okay.

Something that simple could mean so much to them.

And you.

48.

No, This isn't Assisted Suicide

The documentary, "*Living and Dying: A Love Story*" (Share Wisdom Network), is an account and sequence of events, leading up to an elderly couple taking their own lives together, at the same time, with the assistance of a drug prescribed by a physician. They decided that they wanted to be the ones to determine when and where they died, and to be sure to at each other's side when it occurred. Neither wanted to be living alone without the other partner.

Jack Kevorkian was a medical doctor who helped over 130 patients with terminal illnesses, assisting them with methods of taking their own lives to prevent prolonged misery and indignity.

There are countries and some states in the U.S. that have approved assisted suicide under certain conditions.

Some people are for it. Some are against it.

How to care for the elderly, the physically disabled and the terminally ill, is a whole subject in itself. Doctors know how to operate, take out and exchange organs, sew in stitches, set bones and give medications. But they are not necessarily taught much about the philosophical options for people at the end of life.

Does the 92-year-old widowed grandma, who will never walk again, want to try the proposed medical solution, which has a 3% chance of lengthening her life somewhat, but where she'll also have to endure all of the anesthesia, operations and chemo/radiation treatments afterwards, which will then cause her intense pain and unconsciousness for extended periods?

Or, does she want to spend the rest of her days in a comfortable, quiet place, under gentle hospice care and pain management where she can visit with her children, grandchildren and family?

Which choice would you make for her? If you don't do the operations, which may or may not work, is that considered assisted suicide?

There have been some recent studies into this. People are continually revamping care of the elderly to make it gentler, more humane and relevant.

Possibly, further research and compilation will continue to occur to create advanced training and orientation of skills regarding how to negotiate options for those at the end of life, so as to maintain the highest quality of life for an individual, for as long as possible.

It is becoming evident that often, harsh operations, drugs and procedures near the end, even though there is a slim chance of giving a bit more "earth time", destroys the actual quality of life and consciousness of the patient to the point that it's the wrong solution when all is said and done.

The information here is designed to increase the quality of life now, and for however long the person has left. I have actually seen some people who have received one or more of these simple steps, recover to the point of extending their life past the time the doctors thought possible. No claims are made here but it has happened.

More often than not, at some point of using these directives, you'll see resurgence in the dying person. They'll become more aware, their communication increases, there is a bit of time they can say goodbye properly and then within a few hours or day or so later, they pass away peacefully.

You can provide a calmer, less painful place for your loved one, so that it becomes easier for them to let go and move on when the time comes.

49.

It's Not About You

Confronting death is not an easy thing. Our own upsets and losses smack us in the face when dealing with someone at the end of life, especially if it is a family member or loved one.

There is an aspect to all this that I feel you should be made aware of. A person at the end of life often has a hard time understanding why the people around them are so upset.

Keep in mind what it may be like for them. They are lying there in the bed with their own overwhelming situation, wondering what is going to happen, possibly in pain and loss, while at the same time having to deal with a bunch of people around them who are crying, upset and hopeless.

Don't put them in a position of having to counsel you. They've got enough to deal with without having to comfort everyone else.

I recall a woman who was in intensive care for weeks. She had a terminal illness; a breathing device was attached to her face, forcing oxygen into her lungs, and there was little hope for any prolonged future. She was on a morphine drip and had been in and out of consciousness for some time.

At one point, when her husband was at the bedside staring at her in this horrible ICU setting and weary under the intense stress and weeks of coping with it all, he suddenly broke down and started weeping.

His wife suddenly opened her eyes, looked at her husband, pulled off the breathing mask, and in an annoyed, confused tone, blurted out, *"Why are you crying?!"*

Of course, you shouldn't pretend that all is okay when it's not. That would also cause undue stress on the person who is dying. They can sense inauthenticity just like anyone else can.

The appropriate emotion to the scene is fine. Just try limiting an excessive display of overwhelm of your own personal loss, problems and upset. The dying person has a hard-enough time with their own situation, let alone having to try and comprehend what you're going through.

There have been many instances of a dying person hanging on just because they didn't want to create an upset for those they love.

Be real with reassurance and compassion. Not worry and despair.

50.

Denial

We do not want to look at death because it appears it is possibly the complete end of all consciousness and existence. This goes for the person dying and all the others around him or her. It is a hard truth.

They may be not be accepting of the fact their body is dying and they do not want to acknowledge that this reality is possible. In this case, you can say something like, *"Grandpa, in the possibility that this body situation doesn't turn around, I want to know what you need me to take care of that you have your attention on right now"*.

There is a model called "The Stages of Grief" which is detailed in the groundbreaking book by Elisabeth Kübler-Ross M.D., called *"On Death and Dying*.

You may have to deal with people at these various stages of the dying cycle.

These are the emotions people go through when confronted with impending death. It can be studied on its own. Here are the stages:

- Shock & Denial
- Pain & Guilt

- Anger & Bargaining
- Depression, Reflection, Loneliness
- The Upward Turn
- Reconstruction & Working Through
- Acceptance & Hope

Everyone involved will probably be somewhere on this scale at various times around the dying individual. Be aware of this, and on any given day, try to assess where people are at on this list. Then proceed accordingly.

The person at the end of life will most likely go through some of these stages. Even "the upward turn" is a well-known phenomenon that has been observed in people who are dying. The previously terminally ill, incoherent and silent person all of a sudden seems to have a resurgence. He or she starts talking, eating better and seems more energetic. Everyone gets their hopes up that this is a turn-around in the condition, only to find that the next day they're now gone. Dead.

You can bring someone who is dying out of the dark stages of the above scale, and into acceptance and hope. Acceptance that their physical body will eventually perish but with hope for a spiritual future and/or the confidence those that they love will be okay.

51.

Don't Tell the Dying Not to Die

One of the main things you need to remember when counseling or coaching someone is to only ask questions they can answer and only give directions that they possess the ability to carry out. Do not ask or expect anything that is too difficult or impossible, especially those at the end of life. I bring this up because the one thing a dying person can't do anything about is preventing his or her own body death.

You need to let everyone else become aware of this fact. Tell those people around the scene, *"Don't plead or ask (dying person's name) not to die"*. A doctor would never say this to a patient so why would someone else put that burden on them.

Pretty much all these steps and advises are designed to remove fear, anxiety, regret and anything else associated with saying goodbye to everyone and everything he or she has known. This includes the weight of any obligations or duties they may feel they are still responsible for. Giving reassurance that everything will be okay and the permission that it is now all right to depart this life, will help much more than begging them not to die.

Let the dying person know it is okay to let go at any point he or she feels ready.

52.

Environment

Because you are going to be intimately involved in help-ing this dying person with some personal directions and follow-through of their requests, the environment you are assisting them in is one of the first things to address.

Providing a calm, uninterrupted space that you can work together in will help in many ways. Sometimes it is more important than any other step you'll attempt, especially if the surroundings are in a constant turmoil or confusion.

Make attempts to prevent any toxic or aggressive person, family member or staff from agitating the environment around the dying.

Ask people to, *"Please leave the room for a bit, so I can have a moment alone with _____."*

Straighten out any messy items in the room and keep it as clean and orderly as possible. I have noticed that people are apt to bring in lots of pictures and items for the room. They are trying to contribute in any way they can.

Try and keep the clutter to a minimum.

Don't permit inappropriate conversations to occur amongst people in the vicinity of the dying person, as if he or she were not present. Just because they are in a bad way physically and cannot respond as fast as normal, doesn't mean they are not aware. There have been reports of people who had been in deep comas, sometimes under heavy anesthetics, later being able to relay exactly what conversations they heard in the room during the period they were supposedly unconscious.

Respect this fact.

As far as the environment is concerned, I need to mention one last thing. Because emotions tend to be very tense in this situation, there may be family members that complain or get upset at what they perceive as something they feel should or shouldn't be done with regards to their loved one. This frustration is often directed at the staff involved.

You, as the coach, will need to remember and keep in mind what you are there for; to provide comfort and reassurance to the dying person.

This is a delicate scene and needs to be addressed with some thought. Like in life, when you assume people's intentions to be bad, often, it is nothing at all like what you suspected. Many times what is observed as something non-optimum is in reality, an oversight, miscommunication or something not intended.

Jumping down the throat of some nurse, that your grandmother is getting triple-charged for the services she's receiving, and that you will contact a lawyer, and how could you... blah-blah-blah, is quite embarrassing when it turns out there was a glitch in the network, due to a virus in the hospital's billing application, and that this is the first time anyone has been aware of it.

Best to assume that everyone involved is there to help and his or her intentions are good, not harmful. Misguided emotion will create more stress and ill will than anything else.

One client I know observed her elderly father getting worse and worse when she visited him in the hospital. He seemed to be out-of-it more and more each day and his words started slurring incoherently.

She calmly mentioned this observation to her mother, who then went to the doctor and asked to look at her husband's medication chart. In total, he was being given 27 different medications. The doctor realized that this was incorrect and needed to be adjusted. He proceeded to eliminate most of them.

Her father returned to his normal condition and was able to communicate again as usual.

This is the correct way to address that type of situation.

Urge others to bring their concerns, in a polite manner, to the attention of the correct person, so as not to create more confusion to the environment in which you are assisting.

53.

Talk Relay

You may be in a situation where the person you are trying to help can't speak verbally, maybe because of air restrictions, tubes, breathing devices or being in a coma. In these cases, an agreed upon talk relay system can be employed so that you both can maintain a communication line between you.

I once spoke with a speech therapist who said she has used a white board with letters of the alphabet on it and told the patient, who couldn't speak verbally, to *"tap your index finger when I hit the right alphabet letter"*. She also has seen "eye blinks" utilized for the same purpose when the patient was paralyzed and couldn't move any other body part.

People in comas have been known to be able to squeeze the coach's hand as a communication relay. *"Squeeze my hand once for "no" and twice for "yes"* has sometimes worked as a way to inform the coach that his or her actions and words are being understood.

As I've said elsewhere, just because a person can't respond in a normal way, doesn't mean they can't understand you and what is going on. Even if they can speak, a person in physical pain, on medications or at the end of life, will have a response time that is going to be slower than normal, and you'll need to take that into account. If they are answering a question, wait a moment before you speak to ensure they have said all they want to say.

I remember my own grandfather talking to me when he was near the end of his life. He was in a nursing facility and he was quite unhappy about his situation. He said to me, *"They think I don't understand, but I do. I just can't respond as quickly."*

Even though they might appear to be out of it, you'd be amazed at how much an older person is aware of their environment and the things around them.

Use whatever communication system you can develop with the person you are helping, so you two can be in sync with each other when applying these steps. An on-board nurse or speech therapist may have an idea of what method might work best.

54.

Dream On

There is something you should be aware of when it comes to the realities of caring for someone who is dying. This is not listed in the Paranormal Section of this book because it is a different aspect of what you may hear or experience when administering the steps outlined herein.

Those near the end of life may describe to you dreams they are having, where they are seeing and communicating with deceased family members and acquaintances from their past.

Dr. Christopher Kerr interviewed over 1,400 people who were near the end of their lives. He explains and details what he heard from them in the TedX talk I mentioned earlier.

Apparently, these types of pre-death dreams and visions are a common occurrence and need to be acknowledged and dealt with in the correct manner.

Dreams could be said to be a method of processing and orienting ourselves to the various persons and events that have presented themselves to us in our lives. Though many times our dreams seem confusing and random, they often provide insight into situations that we have been trying to figure out analytically.

Sometimes problems get sorted out in our dreams. Other times, we are able to finally face the actual, true intentions, which we buried deep in our subconscious. The realities that we have been pushing away, covering up and hiding behind with the use of social justifications during the normal course of living.

A large percentage of individuals at the end-of-life have been known to talk about the dreams they had, many of which provided them with great comfort and closure.

They have mentioned seeing and communicating with deceased mothers, fathers, siblings, children and friends. The messages they reported receiving were those of harmony, forgiveness and love. They claimed to have finally sorted out past upsets and traumas. The results of their dreams provided them a positive emotional state of peace and dignity.

Dr. Kerr also pointed out that these patients were not confused or disoriented. They were very sequitur in detailing their dreams and spoke with a calmness and serenity. Though their terminal physical condition couldn't be cured, many past spiritual wounds could be resolved through these dreams. Since your purpose is to help another person die with peace and dignity, listening to, acknowledging and validating what their visions mean to them, will help you accomplish what you are there for. Peace, comfort and alleviating fear through dreams, seems to be a fundamental survival mechanism that we apparently all possess. Inform others of this phenomena and allow it to run its course in those you are helping.

55.

The Funeral or Memorial

You may be called on to speak at the service after the person has passed away. Do it.

You'll have a different perspective than other people. You have spent some intimate, truthful moments with the now deceased.

What you have to say could possibly benefit everyone involved.

56.

Don't Feel Guilty

If you feel some relief when someone dies, stop with the guilty feelings.

It's weird. There appear to be these "appropriate reactions" that we all seem to have set-up in life and tacitly agreed on. In other words, how we are supposed to feel, based on particular events. Like the reactions that are deemed socially acceptable when there is a loss, or the ways we are expected to act during a wedding, funeral or graduation.

But then there is the way we actually feel.

The woman, who has given up pretty much everything to care for her sick husband over the last 3 years, is probably going to experience a bit of relief when that burden of worry is over.

Sorry.

The man who is juggling his work, the family finances, his kids' activities and school work, while at the same time also has to deal with his terminally ill wife, going through months of endless cancer operations, chemo treatments, chemo side effects, intensive care stints, relapses and inevitable death, may not be experiencing the same emotions after the funeral that others are feeling.

The 10-year-old who can't play with his friends after school, because he must go visit grandma in the hospital several days a week, isn't going to miss not playing with his friends when she has passed away.

How you handle loss is different than how others may deal with it.

Don't worry if you don't feel how you think others expect you to feel. We grieve in the way we grieve. We all have different relationships, backstories and interactions with the now deceased, so feel what you feel and be okay with it.

If you have been through an extended period of someone you love going through a long and arduous illness, you may have a sense of relief, not only for yourself but for your loved one. *"He doesn't have to suffer anymore"*, *"She is in a better place now"*, are typical phrases spoken after such an ordeal.

The end of one thing is the beginning for something new; don't be too hard on yourself.

Have you ever wondered why there is such uncontrollable grief in adults when their pet dies? For years, I have seen this in my private practice. The emotions and grief people experience, describing seeing their grandma pass away, is nowhere near the torrent of sobbing and tears displayed when they are describing having to go to the vet to put down their dog, Tippy.

In addition to the loss and void of presence now in our home, feelings of failure to help the animal weigh heavily in our hearts.

Finally, I do need to mention one other thing. In the case of the death of a child, there is a dynamic at hand that you should be aware of. Losing a parent, partner, grandparent or friend is one thing.

But losing a child is a different story.

When you are responsible for the upbringing and well being of another human being, and now that entity has died, there is a factor that could be described in the category of "prevention of, or failure to help". This can be extremely devastating to a person. The pain created for this is impossible to describe. A parent is the one in charge of ensuring their children live, so the death of a child brings about not only the attended loss, but also the overwhelming feeling of failure to have helped their child.

The reality regarding the cause of a person's death is rarely someone's "fault", but this will never stop people from going into deep despair over what they imagine they could have done or should have done differently to prevent it. It almost seems to go on automatic. Regret, blaming self and a variety of horrible conceptual scenarios will be going through the minds of those that have lost a loved one, especially a parent losing a child.

You will never know the pain someone else is going through regarding his or her loss. If you notice someone who is feeling guilt or self-blame regarding another's death, maybe these words can shed some light on what's behind it all.

57.

They're Gone. Now What?

After the loved one has passed, there will be some who will be stuck in heavy grief and loss. If there were family members who acted as caretakers for an extended period, there will also be a void of purpose, now that they no longer have that person to care for.

I have seen devastation in the life of one woman whose mother was dying, and her husband also fell ill. She was caring for them both over a longish period of time. Then, in close to the same week, they both suddenly passed away. Her mother and her husband were now gone, and not only was there a huge loss of her loved ones, she also lost a very significant purpose in her life. Caring for the both of them.

There are some simple steps that can be applied to those individuals, to help them get through the grieving process and return to life once again. I have seen some life changing gains in the clients I have helped with grief counseling. It's the kind of thing you don't even know is holding you down until that burden has been lifted.

After the memorial or funeral, if needed, seek out a competent grief counselor for yourself and anybody else in need of some relief.

Section Eight

WORDS OF LOVE

*"Everything will be alright in the end.
If it's not alright, then it's not the end."*

(Anonymous)

58.

I Just Want to Live While I'm Alive

Most of this book refers to helping someone get through the process of body death as peacefully as possible.

But this last section is about you, living your life now. A crash course on a way to look at and live the years you have remaining.

For starters, I compiled a few life regrets and life advices, as told by elderly individuals, some of which were 100 years or older:

- *"Even if you feel hatred, keep it to yourself. Don't hurt other people for any reason."*
- *"Nobody else controls you."*
- *"Love people. Find something to like about the person — it's there — because we're all just people."*
- *"I like to be around positive people, people who lift you up not bring you down."*
- *"I wish I had followed my passion in life."*
- *"I wish I'd cared less about what other people think."*
- *"I wish I had trusted my gut rather than listening to everyone else."*

- *"I wish I hadn't worried so much."*
- *"When you think negatively, you're putting poison on your body."*
- *"Where you're going isn't as important as where you are right now."*
- *"Don't waste your time worrying about getting old."*

Looks like love, caring, being positive and staying true to your own integrity, are the main themes throughout these advices.

Even in the comedy movie, "Defending Your Life", the message is clear. When you're alive, going for your goals, not living in fear and being true to yourself, is the only way you'll be allowed to "move on in the universe" after you die.

We all claim that we want happiness in life. So why are some people constantly so unhappy?

In all my years of coaching and counseling, with everything I have witnessed and learned from all the incredible people I have worked with, with all the materials I have read and all the professionals I have conversed with, everything seems to point to the fact that there seems to be an underlying reason for us to continually possess unpleasant emotions and/or continued bad conditions in our lives.

This is a brutal reality regarding the human condition. You might not like it. Some will hopefully embrace it. Others may throw this book against the wall in protest.

Musician, Willie Nelson has been quoted as saying; *"We*

create our own unhappiness. The purpose of suffering is to help us understand we are the ones who cause it."

Misery can actually become like an addiction. People will look for things to be miserable about in order to feed their desire for unhappiness. There is even a song in the play "Wicked" called "What Is This Feeling?" which contains the lyric; *"There's a strange exhilaration in such total detestation"*.

Emotions we feel stuck in, such as hate, resentment, upset, regret, feelings of victimization, betrayal, anxiety, depression, worry, doubt, fear, as well as constant "bad luck", a lingering illness or a persisting complaint, is often "serving" us somehow. We apparently have some often-forgotten, underlying reason or purpose for having that bad emotion or situation.

Sorry.

It may be an unconscious purpose or an old decision we forgot we made, but it looks like when everything is all said and done, evidence points to the fact that we have something to do with the state of existence we find ourselves in. Good and bad.

Doctors I've met have verified this. Some patients just won't improve or get better, no matter what treatments are administered.

I have actually seen some pretty remarkable recoveries based on this theory. Here are a few examples:

A woman I was once speaking with told me she had a bad jaw problem that had been hurting her for weeks. She had been to dentists, TMJ specialists and orthodontists. Nothing seemed to resolve her pain or jaw misalignment. She was getting pretty hopeless due to the continuous discomfort she was in and the apparent lack of any workable resolution.

I eventually began explaining and talking with her about the fact that people sometimes have an overriding purpose behind a persisting illness or body problem.

Suddenly, right in the middle one of my sentences, her face got flushed, her eyes widened, and she blurted out: "*I know my purpose! I have been yelling at my children too much lately and I just don't want to do that anymore! Oh my god!*"

The next day she told me the jaw pain was gone and she hasn't spoken of it since.

Apparently creating a stiff jaw condition was a solution to the problem of her yelling at her children. It's hard to yell when you can't open your mouth!

* * *

Another example is a man who was frantically telling me how bad his wife was. He was going on and on about how mean she was to him, how she's such a nag, horrible with the kids, our marriage is over, we need a divorce, and how messed-up she is.

I asked him what secrets he had that she didn't know about.

Boom! All the harsh vilifying of his wife stopped immediately.

He sheepishly confided that he had gotten involved with another woman and was freaking out over how to end it. He felt horrible about it and couldn't believe the mess he'd created. He started crying, saying that he really loved his wife and kids but didn't know what to do now.

Selling everyone (and himself) on how bad his wife was made him feel less guilty for what he had done. As long as she was "a no good so and so", whatever immoral acts he'd taken part in could now be rationalized. His situation of having a "bad wife and bad marriage" was used as a purpose for lessening his feelings of guilt. When the truth came out, he no longer had to perpetuate and carry around that self-created condition.

* * *

One executive I was coaching was having a hard time with finances because of the low income being generated and collected at her company. After several attempts at logical plans failing to resolve her problem, I finally asked her something like, "*Is there some underlying reason or purpose you might have for not making money?*"

She thought it over for a bit and then suddenly remembered a weird decision she had made years ago, when she was in her teens. She said that her father was wealthy but very oppressive to her. He would constantly reprimand her for anything she was doing that was not aligned to her becoming a financial success in life. He would belittle any of her actions or activities if he felt it wouldn't add up to her becoming financially stable. They would fight all the time. He'd verbally pound in her, "*You have to make money!*"

And here we go... "Not making money" became the solution to prevent her father from being right! Subconsciously she'd decided if she did well financially then her father would be right, and she'd be wrong. So, in order to get out from under the rule of her father's assertions, she apparently concluded that being broke would be best answer.

After that epiphany about her dad and her decision to stay poor, all of a sudden our coaching plans and programs started working and she became financially solvent and has remained so to this day.

* * *

Another example of this type of phenomena has to do with a psychologist I know. She has a private practice as a counselor and also volunteers for the Red Cross.

Sounds admirable, and it is, but in her home and at social settings, she is constantly remarking and complaining about how bad and dangerous the world is. She talks about children getting abducted, kids getting killed, school shootings, how horrible the government leaders are and how everything is getting destroyed.

She talks like this in front of her own children all the time, and even brings up the idea of killing herself so that her kids will get the insurance money and so hopefully, be able to have a better future to exist in.

Her communication is alarming, frantic, and filled with negativity.

Her children plead with her not to talk like this, but she claims that she loves them and that she is scared for them.

The thing is, she and her family live in a beautiful, million-dollar home, in a very affluent community in one of the safest areas of the country. Her kids are thriving in life. One is at the top of his class academically and the other is in national competitions for gymnastics.

The kids are doing great, but their mother is always painting a gloom-filled picture and fabricates a dangerous environment when it doesn't in fact exist for them in their actual lives.

She says the reason for her out-look is that she is always hearing bad things from her patients and constantly sees the Red Cross reports, so exposure to all this puts her in this state of constant fear for her children.

Wouldn't logic dictate, that if it is true that she really loves her children, but because her profession upsets her so much that she is constantly instilling fear into her kids and denying them the joy of growing up, shouldn't she just quit her job and get a different career?

No, it looks like she has a hidden reason for asserting that the world is bad and dangerous. The two scenarios presented here are contrary to each other. Her family has a great life but then, at the same time, she also claims that her life is dangerous and overwhelming.

One of those two representations is false.

One could only guess as to what underlying reason or purpose she must possess to create the illusion that life is as horrible as she claims it is.

Maybe she feels she has it too good compared to everyone

else she's exposed to, and so must diminish and degrade the life she has. Maybe she feels she has failed to help some of her clients, and therefore, if the world is bad and people are in such a horrible state, any of her failures in helping clients can be justified.

Only she would ultimately be the one to discover her hidden purpose behind painting the world as so awful.

Apparently, that underlying reason or decision is the key motivation behind her actions, even at the expense of her own children's happiness and stability.

* * *

Here are a few main clues to knowing there is an undisclosed purpose or self-serving reason behind someone's bad condition in life:

- There is never any solution that they will propose or accept as workable.
- Your logical suggestions get ignored or worse, demonized.
- Their communication about it gets more and more frantic.
- Their emotions turn on and are asserted harder and harder the more it's discussed.
- Normal treatments don't seem to change it much.

I have always wondered how it is that someone can play a game of football, get physically knocked to the ground and there is no complaint, upset or lingering resentment. Then, that same person could be walking down the street, get knocked down by some whacko in an alley, and all of a sudden, pain, victimization and a huge, overwhelming upset arises.

But it was the same hit. Just a different perception of it.

This is not a popular theory because we all want to think our complaints are "real". They may be on some level, but our emotions and attitudes regarding it can be under our control if we look at it in this different light.

It's like we are subconsciously treating life like a court of law, where we are continually presenting "evidence" to ourselves and others to prove and justify our "case" as to how we are not responsible for why things are the way they are. But there is no judge or jury present to hear our pleading. There's only self-imposed misery in our life and the lives around us.

We will create our own personal disabilities to explain how we are not able to cope with life.

We become a prisoner of our own decisions. When we solve our problems with the wrong solution, that solution becomes the next problem. The little boy pretending to be sick to avoid going to school, may years later develop chronic asthma. The person who cheats on an exam and claims he did it because he's "*not smart enough*", will have a hard time holding a job or moving up in the world due to that asserted decision. The man who justifies his affair by asserting that "*women never show affection*", will eventually have to create for himself a very isolated and lonely life to prove that claim as true.

Making decisions in the middle of a bad or painful situation can affect you for the rest of your life and be a set-up for future trouble.

Love, trust, compassion, serenity and understanding are concepts that can elevate us out of this trap.

Acknowledging what is in front of you, without jumping into a frantic, confused hateful emotion, is a start in leading and experiencing a more enriched life.

Why do people say, "*Count to ten before you react*"? It is so you can back out of the thoughts and emotions that are forced on you by the mind when something bad happens. It also gives you a bigger, more expansive view at what to do or how to proceed with your actions.

Try it next time you feel bad or degrading emotions creep in on yourself. If someone is saying or doing something you disagree with, and you start silently targeting that person as bad, stupid or worse, take a moment and do not react. Just observe what you are feeling and then try to isolate how that unpleasant emotion you're experiencing and that lowered opinion you are developing somehow makes you right. In what way does your position get supported by them being wrong. How does the feeling that they are bad or stupid prove how awesome or righteous you are? How does this build up your own ego?

Gautama Buddha has been quoted as saying, "*Holding onto anger is like grasping a hot coal with the intent of throwing it at someone else; you are the one who gets burned.*"

We have all heard of those top Zen karate masters who rise to a spiritual level where they will never, ever get into a fight with another person. They come to a high-level view of life and do not waste their time getting into how bad or evil another is. They operate from an enlightened understanding of the human condition.

After helping those at the end of life, and the thousands of hours I have spent with individuals coaching and counseling with them, I have seen a pattern that seems to occur with most everyone.

The coaching and counseling sessions I ran were never cut short because of time. We only ended off when a good result occurred. Maybe it took 5 minutes or maybe it took two hours, but the session was terminated when the client hit a point of relief and attained a recognition of some new insight; an improved point of view regarding whatever subject we were addressing. An epiphany, accompanied with a much larger scope than before the session started. A more expansive vision. A less self-opinionated stance of the scene and the personnel involved. More love all around.

Here are a few examples of the types of statements that indicate you have reached the purpose of helping someone in this manner:

- *"Wow, I just realized that my dad had his own struggles and that I've been taking it personally all this time. He was actually just trying to keep it together and figure it all out. I really do love my dad!"*

- *"It just became apparent that whatever I've been accusing others of, I myself have done. I can't continue to fault others like that anymore. What a huge thing to now understand!"*

- *"Now that I look at it, I actually have accomplished so much more than I thought I had. I can stop beating myself up now. Amazing!"*

- (And my favorite) *"Well... it seemed like a good idea at the time."*

Notice, in each case, the person changed their attitude. It was a change in emotion from a negative to a positive.

Where would you rather reside? Negative or positive?

You don't necessarily need a counseling session to come to a more enlighten view of the situations in your life. With a little inspection, you can take yourself out of a negative emotion or aggressive personality and bring yourself to a presence of understanding. Detailed in the book by Byron Katie and Stephen Mitchell, *"Loving What Is: Four Questions That Can Change Your Life*, there is a progressive type of questioning you can do on yourself. If you're feeling victimized, stuck in a bad emotion or anything undesirable that persists, you could ask yourself, *"Who would I be without the thought?"*

There is also a simple, but extremely powerful piece of advice that you should work through and determine how you can apply it in your own life:

"Don't believe everything you think".

I hope you can see by these examples that examining any negative emotion in this way, allows a higher-level look at yourself and the situation you are in, and therefore can pop you out of anything the mind is throwing at you which isn't under your control. Try it next time you feel bad about something.

As I mentioned earlier, people at the end of life will often move into a serene, peaceful, loving perspective. They have accepted "what is" and are no longer fighting to survive. They don't have to prove themselves to anyone on any vector, and so exhibit and pervade the space with a calm understanding of everything.

When the obsession to survive is taken out of the equation, serenity, peace, love and help are possible.

Imagine training yourself to always maintain a high-level view of each life situation you find yourself in. You will still decide and act, but it will be from a much more powerful and stable place. Therefore, things can usually go much better all the way around. In other words, you'll experience more good luck.

Another thought, because this book mostly about providing assistance to someone else, I'll say a few words on that subject.

There is the Latin motto: "*Non nobis solum nati sumus*", which translates to: "Not for us, but for everyone". It means that people should contribute to the general greater good of humanity, apart from working only towards their own interests.

The idea that "we are all connected", is being investigated thoroughly. What you do affects the world around you. How you act, things you try, ideas you hold, all alter and mold your life and the life of others. It is an unavoidable truth.

American author, Gregg Braden, states, "*... experiments in quantum physics, in fact, do show that simply looking at* *something as tiny as an electron – just focusing our awareness upon what it's doing, for even an instance in time – changes its properties while we're watching it. The experiments suggest that the very act of observation is an act of creation."* [10]

You have something to do with the condition of the environment you live in. What you put out there, you will eventually be surrounded by.

The book "Younger Next Year" (Crowley/Lodge), talks about the fact that life and longevity depend a great deal to the degree you stay connected to the world. When people get up in years, they tend to get a bit reclusive, but if you want to stay as youthful and healthy as possible, the best advice is to exercise, eat right, be active and stay connected and committed.

You can accomplish this by continuing to help others. Do everything in your power to make someone's life better.

An important goal we all could strive for, collectively as a species, is an equality of happiness.

59.

Changes

"The only thing that is constant is Change"

(Heraclitus)

Change is a subject that deserves some mention here.

Any upset you have experienced involves a change, to a greater or lesser degree. Especially losing someone or something you love. That type of change can be overwhelming.

Because loss and change seem to be intermingled in our minds, the idea of changing anything is often difficult.

We've seen those people in our lives that have a hard time with change. They stay in a toxic relationship. They won't move to a safer home, in a better location. Some won't break a routine they've done for years because it is "comfortable" the way it is. Some can't even listen to an opposing viewpoint without experiencing anxiety.

When you have lost someone close to you, how to you move on with your life? How do you adjust to that type of upset and change? A parent dies. Your husband or wife has passed away. Even the household pet, you have spent the last 13 years with, had to be put down, and now everything you see around you is a reminder of "how it used to be".

Change = Upset = Stuck in the past.

Life continues. That's for sure. No matter what you are feeling after a loss, life *will* keep going and you'll be part of it.

As far as getting over a bad loss, everyone is different. But there are a couple things to keep in mind. Moving on does not mean forgetting whom you lost. Creating your life with someone new doesn't mean you're replacing anyone.

We will always hold our past loved ones in our hearts and memories. What you experienced and learned, with someone close to you, will always be an integral part of you. That isn't something that gets replaced or forgotten.

When should you start dating again after losing your spouse or life partner? When do you get a new puppy after your old Golden Retriever has died? After your kids have grown and left the house, would becoming a foster parent give a renewed purpose in your life?

Of course, the answer to those questions depends on the person, but realize, there is no rule or acceptable waiting period. Your ability to constantly create your life and maintain communication with the friends, family and world around you, will greatly contribute to your happiness and longevity.

When you have achieved an acceptance of the loss and are ready to continue your life, it is completely okay to embrace it and start again.

60.

A Question of Balance

Weakest Link - *A concept holding that each action in a sequence is dependent upon the performance of the action that came before it. According to the theory, the quality of the series of actions is limited to the quality of the weakest performance in the sequence.*

One piece of advice I once read from someone near the end of life seemed to lean into the concept of a "life balance". He said something along the lines of:

- Take care of your health
- Eat well
- Exercise regularly
- Maintain finances
- Don't fall into the credit trap

Others have advised to maintain a quality of life in areas such as, family, financial, intellectual, social, work, spiritual, recreation, personal growth, romance and more.

The area of life we let slip will eventually pull the rest of it down. The weakest link concept.

It is very unusual that couples that have an awful relationship will wind up being good parents. If you sacrifice your relationship for your children, you have a reasonable chance of losing both.

The executive, who rarely spends time with his family, soon won't have one. The person that overspends will eventually have a lack of money. The woman who puts all her attention to her kids, to the exclusion of the rest of her life, will be totally lost when those children get older and leave the home. Lack of exercise will cause health problems and slow down every other activity. Denying the spiritual side of existence is a denial of self, which holds back imagination, purpose and causation.

I read once that movie director, Oliver Stone, said that his dad told him, "*Everyday do something you don't want to do*". Whatever area of life you are avoiding will eventually become the thing you can no longer escape. It will get to the point where it *must* be dealt with. The thing you're not balancing in your life becomes your weakest link, which then halts the momentum of everything.

List out all the different aspects and areas of your own life and work out a method of keeping everything maintained and coordinated. If needed, find someone who can help you plan it all out and support you in your Life-Balance implementation.

61.

Where is it All Going?

"Life is the dancer and you are the dance"

(Tolle)

Medicine and technology continue to increase the longevity of the lifespan of our human bodies. In 2004 the average age people died was 74 years old. Now, 15 years later in 2019, that age has been increased by 6 years to 79.

Who knows where it's all headed.

With the advancements in technology, we must keep striving for better interpersonal relationships and spiritual well-being across the board.

It should be within all our wishes that the subject called "The Humanities" would see a corresponding positive increase at the same rate as science and technology progress.

Hopefully, coinciding with these improvements, the quality of our lives will continue to improve and the amount of suffering across the planet will decrease proportionally.

The fact that we are all living longer also means that the population is increasing as well. Today there are 7.4 billion people living, eating, breathing, taking up space, being housed, needing meaning, wanting purpose, striving to survive and wondering where it's all going.

With the escalation of the number of humans, comes a greater need to work out the details of how we all can live and prosper together, as humans.

Waiting until someone dies and then realizing you should have told him or her how much you loved them, is a losing proposition. Waiting for a huge catastrophe on this planet, and only then realizing we should have put a greater effort into living in harmony with nature and each other, is the ultimate loss.

In fiction stories and movies, where an alien force is invading earth, the entire planet, with all its inhabitants, races and cultures in every country, come together to fight off these intruders from another galaxy. We all unite to prevent the threat of annihilation.

What if we could all join in a common purpose now and continue like that from here on out?

In my lifetime, I consider the two most major, world-changing events, to have been The Beatles and the Internet.

John Lennon and The Beatles were not only a major catalyst for changing music and art on a worldwide-scale, but they also became the mouthpiece for revolutionary new philosophies such as, "Think for Yourself", "All You Need is Love" and "Give Peace a Chance".

The Internet, along with Google, Facebook and smart phones, has created the ability for the world to communicate with one another instantly. However, the full potential of the Internet, for the good of humanity, has not yet been realized.

What will be the next major event that will change the world? I don't know. We can only speculate. My thought is, the only place it seems that it *should* go is the space that brings science and spirituality together.

The reason artificial intelligence comes across as a scary proposition is because those entities developing A.I. are humans. We've seen what humans can do to each other, so are we really going to be building machines to carry out what *we* want them to do?

Wouldn't it make sense to first try to understand and find answers for questions like, "Where does consciousness come from?" or "What is the human soul?"

"The day when science begins to study non-physical phenomena, it will make more progress in one decade than in all the previous centuries of its existence". (Nikola Tesla)

You get the point.

I know it is human nature for us to create our own problems so we can have something to solve, and there will always be challenges to overcome, but at this point, it appears that the last untapped arena of life, is the "being" part of the composite known as human being. We know what a human is, but what defines "being" or "the being"?

Until that next big event occurs on this planet, maybe we can just engage in helping each other, one on one.

We all have such a short time in these bodies.   An

abbreviated existence. Helping an individual at the end of his or her life really wakes one up to the fact that you have a very brief amount of time to be alive.

Karma is an interesting word. It means (in Hinduism and Buddhism): "*The sum of a person's actions in this and previous states of existence, viewed as deciding their fate in future existences*".

The derivation comes from a Sanskrit word, Karman → action – effect - fate.

In other words, the *action* you put into motion now, and the *effect* that gets created as a result, determines your *fate* later.

Seeing life from the vantage point of someone who is about to pass away is also a good place to get a realistic overview of what is and what is not important in life.

Helping others will keep you connected to life. Teaching others what you have learned, forwards your knowledge to add to a better world. The smallest contribution on your part may result in life changing wisdom for someone else.

I don't know about you, but there have been a few times where someone has reminded me of something I'd said or done that they claimed helped them in their life. And I don't even remember doing or saying it.

You never know when an action or message of yours is going to be something that affects another in a life- changing way.

Whether you're providing aid to someone at the end of

life, middle-of-life or beginning-of-life, it makes for better life all the way around.

A friend once told me that he saw an article that explained how someone had researched and compiled a years' worth of obituaries found in newspapers.

Of course, these types of announcements are normally writings and descriptions of the most positive aspects of people and the lives they lived. Details about their accomplishments, personal loves and pretty much a statement of the best characteristics of an individual are what you'll read in your local periodical regarding people who are now deceased.

A search was then done, through all these collected obituaries, as to which word was most often used in describing these admirable qualities and characteristics of all those people over their lifetimes.

The results showed that the one word used most often was "*help*".

Apparently, what is viewed as most admirable for us as human beings, are the activities of helping one another.

"*Time is your most precious resource. Make every minute count.*" (Brian Tracy)

And when you also make every minute count for the person next to you, that's when you'll *really* know it counts.

62.

And in the End

"I would rather have questions that can't be answered
than answers that can't be questioned."

(Richard Feynman)

When you are helping someone who is dying, remember the concept of "Spirit - Mind – Body". The spirit you are helping now, is the same spirit that was playing in their yard or home when their body was a little kid.

What happens to that spirit when its body has ceased to exist is anybody's guess, belief or faith.

And maybe it will always be that way.

In any game there must be unknowns and barriers otherwise it isn't a game. If you knew every move your chess opponent was going to make, you'd win every time. No game. If you embarked on an adventure, but you were aware of everything that was going to happen around every corner, it would not be an adventure. If you understood exactly how the magician did his tricks, there would be no magic. If you already had every answer there is in life, you would no longer have any desire to ask questions or learn. No motivation. No life.

An answer is a *Stop*. The question is the *Start*. When you find the answer to a question, that is the end of that particular cycle. If we all found the exact answer to the question, "*What is the purpose of life?*" it all might stop.

Life might come to an end.

So, maybe the answer to that question *is* the question.

What if that's the set-up for us all? An arrangement that always provides a curiosity, a hope and therefore a continuation of life.

Maybe those types of deeper questions are not designed to be answered but only to be asked and contemplated, and in that way, this Game of Life will keep on keepin' on.

What is the purpose of life? Maybe to help someone who is dying and then help someone who is living.

Wouldn't you agree that those are a couple worthwhile purposes?

Hope so.

About the Author... me

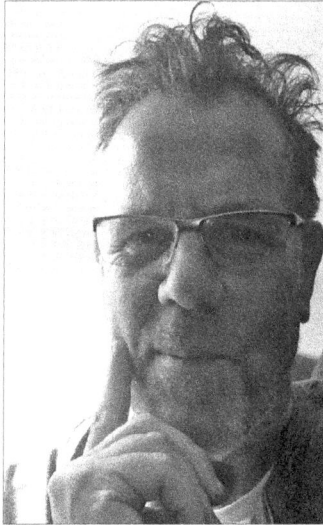

2nd grade - Sitting in class, thinking, *"What am I doing here? What is the point to all this? Am I the only one thinking this stuff?"*

3rd grade - Dad teaches me three chords on a ukulele and I perform a cowboy song, solo, at the school talent show.

4th grade - The Beatles appear on American television for the first time = *"I want to do that!"*

5th grade on... Learned guitar, bass and piano, got into bands, wrote and recorded songs, toured the USA and Japan, made no money ever, met tons of great friends and created lots of awesome memories.

After high school - Worked for a construction company, learned how to build houses, ran a framing crew and became competent at approaching things in a systematic and problem-solving way.

1977 - Drove my motorcycle from Michigan to LA, studied philosophy, various religions, Eastern theology, and new age subjects, including coaching/counseling techniques.

Discovered that giving advice is limited in workability, but by knowing the right question, you can immediately be effective at helping another person in a systematic and problem-solving way.

Mid 1980's on... Started a private coaching/counseling practice in Chicago, (now in California), helping individuals, business owners and couples enhance their lives.

Late 1990's - Developed and refined some steps which help people at the end of life die with peace, dignity and transition to... and coached clients and friends on how to apply those steps to their loved ones.

2019 - Wrote this book.

Contact Rich at:

Email: rich@aboveitall360.com

Website: www.aboveitall360.com

Bibliography

Books:

Kubler-Ross, Elisabeth - *On Death and Dying* - New York, NY - Scribner- 1969

Gawande, Atul - *Being Mortal* - New York, NY - Henry Holt and Company - 2014

Terry Sidford - One Hundred Hearts - Bloomington, Indiana - Balboa Press - 2015

Alexander, Eben - *Proof of Heaven* - New York, NY - Simon & Schuster - 2013

Tolle, Eckhart - *The Power of Now* - London, England - Hodder & Stoughton - 2001

Crowley, Chris - Lodge, Henry - *Younger Next Year* - New York, NY / United Kingdom - Workman Publishing - 2007

Katie, Byron - Mitchell, Stephen - *Loving What Is: Four Questions That Can Change Your Life* - New York, NY, Random House - 2011

Sitchin, Zecharia - *The 12th Planet* - New York, NY / Japan - Ishi Press - 1976

Websites

[1] https://www.statista.com/statistics/274513/life-expectancy-in-north-america/

[2] https://www.hinduwebsite.com/hinduism/h_death.asp

[3] https://en.oxforddictionaries.com/definition/bardo

[4] https://www.caregiverstress.com/geriatric-professional-resources/professional-develoP.M.ent/3ways-to-balance-empathy-with-professional-distance/

[5] https://www.ndtv.com/offbeat/90-year-old-from-texas-says-sorry-for-stealing-stop-sign-from-midvale-utah-75-years-ago-1872143

[6] https://www.express.co.uk/news/science/738387/Time-NOT-real-EVERYTHING-happens-same-time-einstein

[7] https://theconversationproject.org

[8] https://www.historicmysteries.com/the-21-gram-soul-theory/

[9] https://themindsjournal.com/souls-choose-parents-families/

[10] https://allthatsinteresting.com/anunnaki

[11] http://www.superconsciousness.com/topics/science/we-are-all-connected

www.ingramcontent.com/pod-product-compliance
Lightning Source LLC
Chambersburg PA
CBHW052128270326
41930CB00012B/2799